Bacon - Bread   eggs   Wednesday's
 100   120   76 = 3.80
─────────────────────────────
CornFlakes 250 ‖ Dinner   500 ⊦ 1130
─────────────────────────────
                ½ oz
Fat grams Bacon = 2 Bread = 2 eggs = 12

LYNN SONBERG is a book producer and
writer with a special interest in health and
nutrition. She is the author of *The Quick and
Easy Cholesterol and Calorie Counter*, *The
Dietary Fiber Counter to Brand Name and
Whole Foods* and author and co-producer of
The Food Book. In addition she has produced
numerous healthy cookbooks and medical
books including *The All-Natural Sugar Free
Dessert Cookbook*, *Quick and Easy Recipes to
Boost Your Immune System*, *Quick and Easy
Recipes to Lower Your Cholesterol*, *Relief from
Chronic Arthritis Pain*, *Relief from Chronic
Backache* and *What Women Should Know
About Menopause*. She lives and has offices in
New York City.

                        cal
apple Large   51
Banana   105
grapes ½ cup 29
Orange Med.   65
Peach   37
Pear   98
Black Berries ──
   ½ cup   37

egg ──── 76

Bread 1 slice ─ 70

THE QUICK AND EASY FAT GRAM & CALORIE COUNTER

LYNN SONBERG

A LYNN SONBERG BOOK

AVON BOOKS 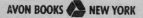 NEW YORK

THE QUICK AND EASY FAT GRAM & CALORIE COUNTER is an original publication of Avon Books. This work has never before appeared in book form.

Research about the health consequences of dietary fat are ongoing and subject to interpretation. Although every effort has been made to include the most up-to-date and accurate information in this book, there can be no guarantee that what we know about this complex subject won't change with time. Readers should bear in mind that this book should not be used for self-diagnosis or self-treatment and should consult appropriate medical professionals before making any major changes in their diet.

AVON BOOKS
A division of
The Hearst Corporation
1350 Avenue of the Americas
New York, New York 10019

Copyright © 1992 by Lynn Sonberg
Published by arrangement with Lynn Sonberg Book Services
Library of Congress Catalog Card Number: 91-92996
ISBN: 0-380-76425-3

First Avon Books Printing: February 1992

AVON TRADEMARK REG. U.S. PAT. OFF. AND IN OTHER COUNTRIES, MARCA REGISTRADA, HECHO EN CANADA.

Printed in Canada.

UNV 10 9 8 7 6 5 4

ACKNOWLEDGMENTS

Special thanks are due to Shelagh Masline for her invaluable help in researching this book and in tracking down especially difficult to find nutrient information. I am also grateful to Lisa Rojak for her contributions.

CONTENTS

INTRODUCTION

WHY ALL THE FUSS ABOUT FAT?

Fats, in the last several decades, have garnered a reputation as the "bad guys" of nutrition.

And rightly so. Americans eat too much fat. All foods are made up of various combinations of fats, proteins, and carbohydrates. And while we need all three basic food components to be well nourished, fats pack more than twice the calories into every gram than either protein or carbohydrates. In addition, one calorie of fat is much harder for the body to burn off than a calorie of either carbohydrate or protein. All of this means that fat in your food means fat on *you*. That's bad enough, but the news gets even worse. Eating too much fat has been shown to increase your risk of heart disease and some forms of cancer. On the other hand, cutting down on fats will provide you with more energy, a slimmer waistline, and overall better health.

You do need *some* fat in your diet to maintain good health, however. Fat is an essential nutrient found in both animal and plant foods. Dietary fats help you to absorb vitamins A, D, E, and K, commonly called the *fat-soluble* vitamins, because they require some fat to be present before the body can utilize them. And since it takes longer for the body to digest fat, a bit of fat at every meal keeps you fuller longer, which helps you resist the temptation to binge on between-meal snacks. Too little fat in the diet can damage your looks, making hair and nails brittle, and drying out your skin.

1

But most people have to worry about eating too much fat, not too little. Most experts, including the American Heart Association and the National Cancer Institute, recommend you get no more than 30 percent of your daily calories from fat. Currently Americans get an average of almost 40 and as much as 60 percent of their calories from fat. Some authorities have advised that people should cut their fat intake to 20 percent of calories. Others even recommend 10 percent of calories, but this is a figure that is extremely difficult for most people to stick to. Besides, most people will improve their cardiovascular health and lose weight simply by reducing their fat intake to the 30 percent level, though some convincing studies indicate that there are additional health benefits from reducing intake even further.

WHY YOU NEED THIS BOOK

Up until now, the problem for most Americans who wish to reduce their fat intake has been how to calculate that 30 percent—or less—every day. This book will do all of the work for you. *The Quick and Easy Fat Gram and Calorie Counter* provides fat gram and calorie counts for 2,500 basic, brand-name, and fast foods. Each listing also tells you what percentage of the food's calories comes from fat. As you'll see in the next section, you no longer have to count calories, but we have provided this information anyway simply because old habits die hard and some readers may still wish to know the caloric value of the foods they eat.

Whether your main goal is a heart-healthy diet, losing weight or simply eating a more nutritious diet, *The Quick and Easy Fat Gram and Calorie Counter* is the only nutrition reference guide you'll ever need.

COUNT FAT GRAMS, NOT CALORIES

Why count fat grams and not calories? Recent studies show that it's the amount of fat you eat, more than calories, that will determine whether you lose or gain weight. Besides, it's easier. Instead of watching your calories, cholesterol, fat, and fiber intake, all you have to do is count your fat grams, and everything else will fall into place. For instance, by reducing your fat intake, you automatically reduce the number of calories and the amount of cholesterol you eat. You'll also automatically increase your intake of foods that are high in fiber and complex carbohydrates, which is the type of diet doctors and major health organizations are promoting today for good health in the nineties. And instead of keeping track of 1,000 to 2,000 calories each day, you'll deal with numbers that range on average from 25 to 70 grams of fat, depending upon your health and weight goals. In short, it's easy to eat a healthy diet by counting fat grams.

Most people will want to count fat grams for the same reasons they counted calories: to lose weight. But whether your concern is losing weight, a healthy heart, cancer prevention, slowing down the aging process, or simply having more energy, controlling your fat intake is the key.

HOW MUCH FAT DO YOU REALLY NEED?

At the bare minimum for good nutrition, an adult man or woman requires only 1 tablespoon or 11 grams of fat each day, which contains only 100 calories. In contrast the average American consumes from 70 to 100 grams of fat, or a whopping 630 to 900 calories from fat each day.

So what should your optimum fat intake be? That depends on your general health and weight-loss goals. Certainly everyone can benefit from reducing fat intake to the 30 percent-of-total-calories level recommended by most major health organizations. Other people may wish to make a more dramatic change. Some health authorities, including the American Health Foundation, recommend reducing fat intake to the 20 percent level. Here's how to figure out what all of this means:

Look at the table below. First find your desired weight in the left-hand column (or your current weight if you are happy with it). Then, to find your daily fat gram quota, choose from one of the four right-hand columns.

- If you simply want to improve your health without making major changes in your eating habits, choose the fat gram quota under the 30 percent column. If you are overweight, chances are that you will lose weight eating this amount of fat.
- If you are interested in more rapid weight loss and/or desire the increased health benefits that some experts believe a lower fat diet can bring, choose the fat gram quota under the 15 or 20 percent column.

Desired Weight	Maintenance Calories	Calories From Fat			
		15%	20%	25%	30%
WOMEN					
100	1,500	25 g	33 g	42 g	50 g
110	1,650	28 g	37 g	46 g	55 g
120	1,800	30 g	40 g	50 g	60 g
130	1,950	33 g	43 g	54 g	65 g
140	2,100	35 g	47 g	58 g	70 g
150	2,250	38 g	50 g	63 g	75 g
160	2,400	40 g	53 g	67 g	80 g
MEN					
135	2,025	34 g	45 g	56 g	68 g
145	2,175	36 g	48 g	60 g	72 g
155	2,325	39 g	52 g	65 g	78 g
165	2,475	41 g	55 g	69 g	83 g
175	2,625	44 g	58 g	73 g	88 g
185	2,775	46 g	62 g	77 g	92 g
195	2,925	49 g	65 g	81 g	98 g

Whichever fat gram level you choose, we recommend a gradual approach. Start at the 30 percent level and after you've become accustomed to this style of eating, gradually reduce your fat intake even more.

A word of warning. It's quite possible to blow your entire daily fat gram quota on a fast-food cheeseburger and fries. On rare occasions there may be no harm in this, but if you make a habit of it, this eating plan is doomed to fail. Instead, learn to relish foods rich in fiber and complex carbohydrates such as pastas, grains, legumes, fruits, and vegetables that are as satisfying as they are healthful. These delicious low-fat foods are the key to effortless weight loss and optimum health.

How exactly do you go about changing to a lower fat style of eating? Beginning on page 11, this book will give you a wealth of practical advice on smart food choices, recipe substitutions, shopping, food preparation, and more. But first let's take a closer look at fats. Just what is it about fat that makes it so destructive to our health?

A CLOSER LOOK AT FATS

Exactly what are fats and how do they operate in your body?

There are three different kinds of dietary fat: saturated, polyunsaturated, and monounsaturated. They are differentiated by their molecular structure according to how many hydrogen atoms each molecule contains. A saturated fat molecule has four out of four possible hydrogen atoms. A monounsaturated fat molecule has one of the four hydrogen positions empty and a polyunsaturated fat molecule has two of the four hydrogen positions empty.

Before we can describe the health effects of these different types of fats, we need to understand something about two other key players in fat metabolism: triglycerides and cholesterol.

Triglycerides

When the body digests fats, it breaks them down into chains of molecules, which then bind together in a form of triplets called *triglycerides*. Triglycerides then flow from the intestines into the lymphatic system until they are dumped into the bloodstream. The greater the amount of triglycerides in the blood, the thicker the blood and the harder the heart has to work to pump this thicker liquid through the blood vessels.

If you eat a diet high in fat you are more likely to develop high triglyceride levels. A high sugar diet is also a risk factor for developing high triglycerides for approximately 20 million Americans.

Cholesterol

Cholesterol is a fatty waxlike substance that our bodies need in order to function. It is manufactured in the body and used, for example, to manufacture substances in our cell membranes and nerves. Although we don't actually need any cholesterol at all in the diet after the first six months of life, most Americans consume excessive amounts of this substance (which is only present in foods of animal origin), which results in high blood cholesterol levels, especially in the presence of too much saturated fat. When blood cholesterol is high, it can cling to the arterial walls and eventually become hardened with calcium, a condition called *atherosclerosis*, which can lead to heart attacks and strokes.

Cholesterol is transported in molecules called *lipoproteins*. High-density lipoproteins, HDLs, carry cholesterol to the liver where it is excreted and delivered throughout the body for cell metabolism and repair. HDL can help lower serum cholesterol levels. Low-density lipoproteins, LDLs, also carry cholesterol into the bloodstream, but they do not allow the body to use it. Therefore, much of the low-density lipoproteins end up as cholesterol plaque deposits on the walls of the arteries.

Aerobic exercise can help protect against heart disease by raising the level of beneficial HDL cholesterol in the blood.

Saturated Fat

Among all of the fats, saturated fat is the most unhealthy. Too much saturated fat in the diet tends to raise cholesterol levels in the blood and is strongly linked to the high incidence of heart disease among Americans. Many health authorities believe that monitoring saturated fat intake is even more important than monitoring cholesterol intake.

The more saturated a fat is, the more it remains firm at room temperature, an easy way to tell if you're eating saturated fat.

You should also try to avoid "hydrogenated" or "partially hydrogenated" fats and oils. These are basically polyunsaturated vegetable oils that have been chemically altered. Their effect on the body is similar to that of saturated fat.

Some health authorities recommend that you get no more than 10 percent of your calories from saturated fat, or 20 grams per day for someone consuming 1,800 calories a day. Other experts believe this figure is too high and that no more than 10 grams a day of saturated fat is optimal.

Foods high in saturated fat include meats (especially red meats), cheeses, whole milk products, butter, and coconut and palm oils.

Polyunsaturated Fats

Polyunsaturated fats have received a lot of attention because of their ability to lower serum cholesterol levels. That's why you see everything from potato chips to frozen chicken dinners labelled "high in polyunsaturated fats."

There is bad news about polyunsaturates, however. Polyunsaturated fats can damage the body's immune system by producing unstable molecules called *free radicals* during metabolism. When polyunsaturates are heated, the empty spaces in the molecule fill up with oxygen. This oxidation makes the oil turn rancid. When this toxic fat is metabolized, free radicals are released, damaging healthy tissue, accelerating the aging process, and possibly compromising the immune system.

Gram for gram, polyunsaturated fats are still better for you than saturated fats, but you should eat them in moderation. (It's not a good idea to avoid them altogether, however. Polyunsaturated fat is the only source of linoleic acid, an essential fatty acid, so be sure to consume a small amount of polyunsaturated oil each day.) To limit free radical formation, it's best to consume any polyunsaturated oils unheated.

Foods high in polyunsaturated fats include most vegetable oils, fish, almonds, and walnuts.

Monounsaturated Fats

Monounsaturated fats are the healthiest fats to eat. Monounsaturated fats selectively lower the more harmful LDL cholesterol while polyunsaturated fats lower both LDL and HDL cholesterol. Unlike polyunsaturates, the monounsaturated molecule is stable, and therefore not linked to free radical damage.

A recent study from China shows, however, that even too much monounsaturated fat can cause trouble. Researchers from Shanghai Medical University and the National Cancer Institute in Toronto discovered that women who ate a diet moderately low in fat by American standards (containing 34 percent of calories from fat) but high in monounsaturates (70 percent of fat intake was monounsaturated) increased their risk of breast cancer by 20 percent. The study suggests that the risk of breast cancer increases when the quantity of monounsaturated fats in the diet is too great in proportion to other fats.

Foods high in monounsaturated fats include peanuts, olives and their oils, cashews, and avocados.

Fats and Heart Disease

The link between too much fat in the diet and the more than 500,000 American lives lost annually to heart and coronary disease is indisputable. Though our intake of saturated fat and cholesterol has dropped significantly in the last three decades, Americans still eat, on the whole, more fat, including more polyunsaturated fat, than they did a generation ago. Almost without exception, foods rich in cholesterol are also rich in fat. By cutting down on fat consumption, you'll automatically be cutting down on cholesterol.

While this has brought down the total number of heart attacks, it has actually served to increase the number of deaths from cancer. As previously explained, an increased intake of polyunsaturated fats can negatively affect the immune system.

We have been taking steps in the right direction, but unfortunately that's not enough. Cutting down our overall fat consumption is still the key to reducing our risk of becoming a member of the largest statistical group in America.

Fats and Cancer

People who eat a lot of fat tend to be overweight, and obesity has long been associated with increased risk of cancer. If you eat too much fat, you're automatically at risk for contracting two types of frequently fatal cancers: cancer of the colon and of the breast. These cancers occur mostly in countries where a high-fat diet is typical, such as the United States and Scandinavia. These cancers are rare in countries such as Japan and China, but when Orientals move to the United States and start to eat a high-fat diet, their risks of getting colon and breast cancer quickly reach the levels of lifelong Americans.

Why does cancer risk increase? A high-fat diet usually contains a lot of dietary cholesterol. When the cholesterol breaks down in the colon, some of the by-products act like estrogen and other female hormones. These substances stimulate tissue in the breast, which is sensitive to female hormones, and can create tumors and unusual growths.

Also fats move more slowly through the lower intestine than either carbohydrates or protein. When a fatty food stays in the colon longer, more of the harmful substances in the food are absorbed into the system, including those that can cause colon cancer.

Red meat, a food high in saturated fat, was recently singled out in a Boston-based study as a prime cause of colon cancer. The researchers found that women who eat beef, pork, or lamb every day are two and a half times more likely to get colon cancer than women who ate red meat rarely, i.e., less than once a month.

Fats and the Immune System

The immune systems of most Americans may not be operating at peak efficiency, with poor nutrition the most likely culprit. Free radical damage is one factor, as is the fact that a high-fat diet is very likely to be low in nutrition. Overly processed and refined junk foods such as hot dogs, potato chips, and Ring Dings tend to be high in fat and low in the nutrients that boost the immune system, vitamins A, C, and E, zinc, and selenium.

Recent studies have shown that Omega-3 fatty acids may slow down or prevent the spread of cancer cells, increase the number and activity of disease-fighting white blood cells, reduce the level of triglycerides and cholesterol in the blood, and actually prevent the onset of atherosclerosis.

Though fish-oil capsules are now found in health-food and drug stores, some studies have shown that Omega-3 fatty acids, when isolated from natural food sources, are not effective immune boosters.

The best natural sources of Omega-3 fatty acids are most types of fish, especially those high in fat such as salmon, mackerel, and trout—as well as wheat germ oil, dark green vegetables, soybeans, beans, and canola oil.

PRACTICAL TIPS FOR REDUCING FAT IN YOUR DIET

Now that you know why you should cut down your fat intake, here are some practical tips on how to do it.

Increase the Fiber in Your Diet

When you begin to cut down on your intake of fat by counting fat grams, you'll find that the amount of high-fiber foods you eat will naturally increase. Why? You'll have to replace the missing fat with something, and many low-fat foods are naturally high in fiber.

Fiber is a noncaloric, indigestible plant material that fills you up by absorbing water, then helps to eliminate the waste that's left behind from eating foods that are low in fiber. Plant foods are the only source of dietary fiber.

Select high-fiber foods such as whole-grain cereals and breads, fruits and vegetables, and legumes. Foods that are high in fiber and carbohydrates are extremely satisfying, so you may be surprised to find that you don't even miss the fatty foods you used to crave. Another bonus is that high-fiber foods take longer to eat than high-fat foods. This slows down your eating. Since it takes about 20 minutes for the stomach to signal to the brain that it's full, you'll ingest far fewer fiber-filled calories in that time period than if you spent the same amount of time eating fat.

One of the easiest ways to cut down on your fat intake is by substituting low-fat foods for their high-fat counterparts when cooking or baking. In most cases, this can be done without a loss of quality or flavor in the finished product.

Fat Substitutes in Recipes

- Use two egg whites in place of one whole egg and three egg whites instead of two eggs. You'll cut down on cholesterol and fat simultaneously without sacrificing taste or quality.

- Use low-fat ricotta cheese instead of cream cheese.
- Opt for low-fat yogurt instead of sour cream.
- Use vegetable-oil spray instead of butter to grease pans and cookie sheets.
- When a recipe calls for milk, try fruit juice or broth instead, depending on whether the dish is supposed to be sweet or savory. You'll save fat and increase the flavor.
- Instead of using cream to thicken soups and gravies, try adding pureed cooked vegetables, bread crumbs, or even farina.
- Buy one of those measuring cups that separates the fat from the liquid in chicken or beef broth.

The New Fat Substitutes: Do They Work?

In the last few years, several food manufacturers have developed fat substitutes that are added to everything from ice cream to pastries in an effort to persuade Americans that they really *can* have their cake and eat it too.

Unfortunately, preliminary studies have shown that eating a cake made with a fat substitute will not alleviate a craving for a real piece of cake. In addition, the foods made from fat substitutes are almost always highly processed and low in nutrients.

Some nutritionists have commented that indulging in fat substitutes seems to be an invitation to binge on the real thing later on, canceling out all the effort you've made to watch your fat intake.

We recommend you forget about artificial fat substitutes and count fat grams in real food instead with *The Quick and Easy Fat Gram and Calorie Counter*.

More Tips on Low-Fat Eating

- Wean yourself off cream, half-and-half, and other fattening additions to your coffee. Instead try 2-percent milk, which tastes almost as rich. And stay away from the powdered coffee "creamers," which often contain saturated coconut oil.

- Always choose low-fat milk products: low-fat yogurts, cheeses, milk, ice creams. The reduction in fat adds up.

- Instead of having meat and potatoes for dinner, cut up that piece of meat and stir-fry it (using a minimal amount of oil) with those potatoes and other vegetables such as onions, carrots, broccoli, and snow peas. Add a little broth if the food sticks to the pan. You'll reduce your fat intake and increase your intake of complex carbohydrates.

- Use a vegetable-oil spray or brush to oil pans thoroughly, without excess fat. Better yet, use nonstick pans.

- When cooking meat or poultry, use a steamer rack, which will allow the fat to drip away.

- *Always* cut the fat off meat and the skin off chicken before cooking. Cook in a bit of broth to maintain juiciness.

- Instead of cooking vegetables and slathering them with butter, add a few drops of sesame oil or chili oil for flavor without a lot of fat.

- Read ingredients lists and avoid high-fat foods by watching for the words *oil, shortening, lard, hydrogenated*, and *partially hydrogenated oils*. And the higher up on the ingredient list fat appears, the more the product contains.

- When buying meat, choose a grade of Good over Choice or Prime, both of which contain more fat than Good.

- When cooking meat dishes such as stews and roasts, prepare a day ahead, refrigerate, then skim off the hardened fat before reheating. Do the same thing with canned broth.

- Stay away from processed meats such as hot dogs and cold cuts. Even meats that are seemingly low in fat, such as salami and bologna made from turkey instead of beef or pork, still get up to 80 percent of their calories from fat. Choose unprocessed cold cuts such as turkey breast, roast beef, and baked ham. They're a lot lower in sodium, too.

- Low-fat cheeses such as neufchatel and feta are good as well as the new versions of old favorites such as cheddar and Swiss that are made with low-fat milks, but avoid "imitation" cheeses, in which part of the fat has been replaced with vegetable oil, which is sometimes saturated. Since even the low-fat cheeses are still relatively high in fat, use them sparingly.

- Develop a standard repertoire of low-fat dishes you can rely on in a pinch. Then keep most of the staple ingredients in the house.

- Stick to your low-fat shopping list when you go to the supermarket. Develop an iron will that can say no to the three-for-a-dollar high-fat cheese crackers tantalizingly placed at the end of the aisle. If you find they made their way into your cart, picture your arteries and the plaque sticking to them after you eat the cheese crackers and put them back on the shelf.

- Try the new oil-free salad dressings. Or better yet, make your own, from broth, herbs, lemon juice, and garlic.

- Make your own microwave meals instead of buying low-calorie frozen dinners that may be high in fat. Just precook chicken breasts, fish, or lean beef, rice, and vegetable, and place in a reusable microwave container. Add a little defatted broth to the container to maintain moistness during reheating. You'll have a freezer full of ready-made dinners that are lower in fat and cost less than any frozen dinner on the market.

- *Cholesterol-free* doesn't mean *fat-free*. Always read the label for the number of grams of fat per serving, and the ingredient panel for anything with the word *fat* or *oil* on it.

Eating Out

- When you're invited out to a friend's house for dinner, bring your own low-fat casserole, enough for a few people.

- *Never* order anything with the words *fried, sautéed*, or *browned, creamed*, or *buttered* in it. These terms are really sneaky substitutes for the term *high-fat*. Instead, look for entrees that are *roasted, braised, poached, steamed*, and *baked*.

- When you fly, always call ahead 24 hours before flight time to order a vegetarian meal or fruit plate.

- If you haven't already gotten into the habit, *always* ask for salad dressing on the side. And if an entree comes with gravy, tell the waiter to skip it.

- For a low-fat change of pace, order a couple of appetizers such as soup, salad, some bread, and maybe half an order of pasta in tomato-based sauce instead of an entree.

- If you don't see fresh fruit on the dessert tray, ask for it.

- Regularly dine at restaurants that list entrees as "heart-healthy," and tell the manager how much you appreciate it. Ask for low-fat meals at other restaurants.

- When you order a dish to be prepared without fats or oils and it arrives at your table swimming in butter, send it back. And if the chef claims to be insulted, find a restaurant that will give you what you want.

- Many of the habits you've developed over the years from counting calories can be applied to counting fat grams. You've probably had lots of practice. Just add these tips to the ones you already know, and you'll be well on your way to eating healthfully and low-fat.

- Before you eat any food, look it up in *The Quick and Easy Fat Gram and Calorie Counter* to check how much fat it contains. Jot down the number of fat grams you eat each day and try to stay aware of the running total. Carry this book with you wherever you go— shopping, eating out, etc.—to make sure you keep within your daily fat intake allotment.

With *The Quick and Easy Fat Gram and Calorie Counter*, eating healthfully to lose weight is now foolproof. If you are a woman who wants to lose weight quickly, safely, and easily, limit your daily intake of fat to between 30 and 50 grams a day. A man who wants to lose weight should eat foods that range from 40 to 65 grams daily. *For more detailed guidelines, refer to the table on page 4.*

The Quick and Easy Fat Gram and Calorie Counter is your guide to beginning a whole new way of eating. Remember, before making any major change in your diet, consult your physician.

FAT AND CALORIE
COUNTER

ABBREVIATIONS AND SYMBOLS

% . . . . percentage
fl oz . . . . fluid ounce
oz . . . . ounce
pc . . . . piece
tbsp . . . . tablespoon
tsp . . . . teaspoons
Tr . . . . trace amount*
< . . . . less than*

All foods are ready to eat or prepared according to package instructions, unless otherwise specified.

---

* Trace amounts of fat were rounded off to .25 grams, and less than 1 gram fat was rounded off to .5 grams when figuring percentages of calories from fat.

Product	Portion	Calories	Percent Calories from Fat	Fat Grams

BEEF

Note: All figures are for separable lean meat unless otherwise noted.

Product	Portion	Calories	Percent Calories from Fat	Fat Grams
Brain, fried	3 oz	167	70	13
Breakfast strips	2 strips	102	71	8
Breakfast strips (Oscar Mayer)	2 strips	92	78	8
Breakfast strips (Sizzlean)	2 strips	70	64	5
Brisket, braised	3 oz	205	48	11
Brisket, flat half, braised	3 oz	223	52	13
Brisket, point half, braised	3 oz	181	35	7
Chuck, arm pot roast, braised	3 oz	196	37	8
Corned beef	3 oz	213	68	16
Flank steak, braised	3 oz	208	52	12
Flank steak, broiled	3 oz	207	57	13
Hamburger, extra lean, baked, medium	3 oz	213	59	14
Hamburger, extra lean, baked, well-done	3 oz	232	54	14
Hamburger, extra lean, broiled, medium	3 oz	217	58	14
Hamburger, extra lean, fried, medium	3 oz	216	58	14

Product	Portion	Calories	Percent Calories from Fat	Fat Grams

BEEF

Note: All figures are for separable lean meat unless otherwise noted.

Product	Portion	Calories	Percent Calories from Fat	Fat Grams
Hamburger, extra lean, raw	3 oz	259	56	16
Hamburger, lean, baked, medium	3 oz	227	63	16
Hamburger, lean, broiled, medium	3 oz	231	62	16
Hamburger, lean, broiled, well-done	3 oz	238	57	15
Hamburger, lean, fried, medium	3 oz	234	62	16
Hamburger, lean, raw	3 oz	264	58	17
Hamburger, regular, baked, medium	3 oz	244	66	18
Hamburger, regular, broiled, medium	3 oz	246	66	18
Hamburger, regular, fried, medium	3 oz	260	66	19
Hamburger, regular, fried, well-done	3 oz	243	59	16
Hamburger, regular, raw	3 oz	264	58	17
Hamburger (Micro Magic)	1	350	46	18
Kidneys, simmered	3 oz	122	22	3
Liver, fried	3 oz	184	34	7
Porterhouse steak, broiled	3 oz	185	44	9

Product	Portion	Calories	Percent Calories from Fat	Fat Grams

BEEF

Note: All figures are for separable lean meat unless otherwise noted.

Product	Portion	Calories	Percent Calories from Fat	Fat Grams
Pot roast, braised	3 oz	196	37	8
Rib eye, large end, broiled	3 oz	183	49	10
Rib eye, large end, roasted	3 oz	197	50	11
Rib eye, small end, broiled	3 oz	191	47	10
Rib eye, small end, roasted	3 oz	206	52	12
Round, raw	3 oz	114	32	4
Round, broiled	3 oz	157	34	6
Round, bottom, braised	3 oz	182	35	7
Round, eye, roasted	3 oz	151	30	5
Round, tip, roasted	3 oz	156	35	6
Round, top, broiled	3 oz	156	29	5
Short ribs, braised	3 oz	251	53	15
Sirloin steak, broiled	3 oz	170	37	7
T-bone steak, broiled	3 oz	182	45	9
Tenderloin, broiled	3 oz	167	38	7
Tenderloin, roasted	3 oz	177	46	9
Tongue, simmered	3 oz	241	67	18
Top loin, broiled	3 oz	162	33	6
Tripe, raw	3 oz	83	33	3

Product	Portion	Calories	Percent Calories from Fat	Fat Grams

BEVERAGES

BEER

Product	Portion	Calories	Percent Calories from Fat	Fat Grams
Ale	12 fl oz	147	0	0
Beer	12 fl oz	156	0	0
Light beer	12 fl oz	100	0	0

CARBONATED DRINKS

Product	Portion	Calories	Percent Calories from Fat	Fat Grams
Bitter Lemon	12 fl oz	192	0	0
Club soda	12 fl oz	0	0	0
Coca-Cola	12 fl oz	144	0	0
Cream soda	12 fl oz	156	0	0
Diet Coke	12 fl oz	1	0	0
Diet Pepsi	12 fl oz	1	0	0
Diet 7-Up	12 fl oz	4	0	0
Diet Sprite	12 fl oz	4	0	0
Dr. Pepper	12 fl oz	156	0	0
Fresca	12 fl oz	4	0	0
Ginger ale	12 fl oz	113	0	0
Grape soda	12 fl oz	179	0	0
Mountain Dew	12 fl oz	171	0	0
Orange soda	12 fl oz	179	0	0
Pepsi-Cola	12 fl oz	156	0	0
Perrier	12 fl oz	0	0	0
RC Cola	12 fl oz	156	0	0
Root beer	12 fl oz	163	0	0
Seltzer	12 fl oz	0	0	0
7-Up	12 fl oz	144	0	0
Sprite	12 fl oz	144	0	0
TAB	12 fl oz	1	0	0
Vernor's	12 fl oz	139	0	0

COFFEE

Product	Portion	Calories	Percent Calories from Fat	Fat Grams
Brewed	6 fl oz	3	0	0

Product	Portion	Calories	Percent Calories from Fat	Fat Grams

BEVERAGES

COFFEE
Instant	6 fl oz	4	0	0
Cafe Amaretto	6 fl oz	51	53	3
Cafe Amaretto, sugar free	6 fl oz	35	77	3
Cafe Francais	6 fl oz	55	49	3
Cafe Francais, sugar free	6 fl oz	35	51	2
Cafe Irish Creme	6 fl oz	55	49	3
Cafe Irish Creme, sugar free	6 fl oz	30	6	2

DISTILLED LIQUORS
(all varieties)
80 Proof	1 fl oz	65	0	0
90 Proof	1 fl oz	74	0	0
100 Proof	1 fl oz	83	0	0

JUICES: FRUIT/VEGETABLE
Apple, bottled	8 fl oz	116	0	0
Apple, frozen	8 fl oz	111	0	0
Carrot, fresh	8 fl oz	96	0	0
Grape, bottled	8 fl oz	155	0	0
Grapefruit, frozen	8 fl oz	102	0	0
Orange, canned	8 fl oz	104	0	0
Orange, frozen	8 fl oz	112	0	0
Pineapple, canned	8 fl oz	137	0	0
Prune, bottled	8 fl oz	181	0	0
Tomato	8 fl oz	4	0	0

PUNCHES, JUICE DRINKS
Cranberry juice (Ocean Spray)	8 fl oz	147	0	0
Five Alive	8 fl oz	87	0	0

Product	Portion	Calories	Percent Calories from Fat	Fat Grams
BEVERAGES				
PUNCHES, JUICE DRINKS				
Gatorade	8 fl oz	39	0	0
Hawaiian Punch	8 fl oz	89	0	0
Kool-Aid	8 fl oz	98	0	0
Lemonade, frozen	8 fl oz	96	0	0
Tang	8 fl oz	119	0	0
TEA				
Brewed	6 fl oz	0	0	0
Herbal	6 fl oz	0	0	0
Iced, instant	6 fl oz	2	0	0
WINE				
Champagne	4 fl oz	84	0	0
Red	3½ fl oz	76	0	0
Sauternes	3½ fl oz	84	0	0
Sherry	2 fl oz	84	0	0
White	3½ fl oz	80	0	0
BREAD, MUFFINS, AND ROLLS				
BAGELS				
Plain	1	200	9	2
Egg	1	200	9	2
Onion (Sara Lee)	1	250	7	2
Poppy seed (Sara Lee)	1	230	8	1
Sesame seed (Sara Lee)	1	260	10	3
Biscuit	1	100	45	5
Biscuit (Weight Watchers)	1	50	9	<1
Bran'nola	1 slice	70	13	1

Product	Portion	Calories	Percent Calories from Fat	Fat Grams

BREAD, MUFFINS, AND ROLLS

Product	Portion	Calories	Percent Calories from Fat	Fat Grams
Bread crumbs (Contadina)	½ cup	213	8	2
Bread sticks (Stella D'Oro)	2	82	22	2
Brown, canned	1 slice	160	6	1
Cornbread	1 pc	107	17	2
Cinnamon (Pepperidge Farm)	1 slice	85	32	3
Cracked Wheat (Pepperidge Farm)	1 slice	70	13	1
Croissant	1	235	46	12
Dark bread (Hollywood)	1 slice	40	23	1
French bread	1 slice	100	9	1
Honey Wheat Berry (Pepperidge Farm)	1 slice	70	13	1
Italian bread	1 slice	85	11	1
Mixed grain	1 slice	65	14	1
MUFFINS				
Apple Cinnamon Spice (Sara Lee)	1	220	33	8
Blueberry (Pepperidge Farm)	1	170	32	6
Blueberry (Sara Lee)	1	200	36	8
Bran, homemade	1	112	40	5
Corn, homemade	1	126	29	4
English (Pepperidge Farm)	1	140	13	2
Oatmeal	1 slice	65	14	1

Product	Portion	Calories	Percent Calories from Fat	Fat Grams
BREAD, MUFFINS, AND ROLLS				
Pita (Sahara)	1 pocket	65	14	1
Pumpernickel (Arnold)	1 slice	80	11	1
Raisin (Arnold)	1 slice	70	13	1
Raisin Cinnamon (Pepperidge Farm)	1 slice	75	24	2
ROLLS				
Dinner rolls (Roman Meal)	1	45	20	1
Frankfurter (Country Kitchen)	1	120	15	2
Golden Twist (Pepperidge Farm)	1	110	49	6
Hamburger (Pepperidge Farm)	1	130	14	2
Hamburger (Shop 'n Save)	1	120	15	2
Parker House (Pepperidge Farm)	1	60	15	1
Potato (Martin's)	1	130	14	2
Sandwich roll	1	162	17	3
Whole wheat	1	90	10	1
Roman Meal	1 slice	68	13	1
RYE BREADS				
Dill Rye (Arnold)	1 slice	80	11	1
Levy's	1 slice	80	11	1

Product	Portion	Calories	Percent Calories from Fat	Fat Grams
BREAD, MUFFINS, AND ROLLS				
RYE BREADS				
Light (Arnold Bakery)	1 slice	40	11	<1
Party Rye (Pepperidge Farm)	4 slices	60	15	1
Seeded Family Rye (Pepperidge Farm)	1 slice	40	23	1
Stub Pullman Rye (Freihofer's)	1 slice	70	13	1
Seeded Rye (Pepperidge Farm)	1 slice	80	11	1
Seven Grain (Home Pride)	1 slice	70	13	1
WHITE BREADS				
Arnold Brick Oven	1 slice	60	15	1
Country Hearth	1 slice	70	13	1
Freihofer's	1 slice	70	13	1
Fresh Horizons	1 slice	50	18	1
Pepperidge Farm	1 slice	73	18	2
Wonder	1 slice	70	13	1
Wonder, buttermilk	1 slice	70	13	1
WHOLE WHEAT BREADS				
Arnold Brick Oven	1 slice	60	30	2
Arnold Light Golden	1 slice	40	11	<1
Country Hearth	1 slice	70	13	1
Freihofer's	1 slice	75	12	1

Product	Portion	Calories	Percent Calories from Fat	Fat Grams

BREAD, MUFFINS, AND ROLLS

WHOLE WHEAT BREADS

Product	Portion	Calories	Percent Calories from Fat	Fat Grams
Fresh and Natural	1 slice	70	13	1
Fresh Horizons	1 slice	49	2	Tr
Home Pride Butter Top	1 slice	70	13	1
Home Pride Butter Top Light	1 slice	40	11	<1
Home Pride Wheatberry	1 slice	70	13	1
Wheat Germ (Pepperidge Farm)	1 slice	65	7	<1
Whole Wheat (Pepperidge Farm)	1 slice	65	14	1
Wonder	1 slice	70	13	1

CAKE

DESSERT CAKES

Product	Portion	Calories	Percent Calories from Fat	Fat Grams
Angel food, homemade	1/12 cake	161	1	Tr
Angel food, from mix (Duncan Hines)	1/12 cake	131	1	Tr
Banana (Pillsbury)	1/12 cake	250	40	11
Carrot (Duncan Hines)	1/12 cake	187	19	4
Cheesecake (Royal)	1/8 cake	225	36	9
Chocolate, from mix	1/12 cake	250	40	11

Product	Portion	Calories	Percent Calories from Fat	Fat Grams

CAKE

DESSERT CAKES

Product	Portion	Calories	Percent Calories from Fat	Fat Grams
Chocolate Chip (Pillsbury)	1/12 cake	270	47	14
Devil's Food (Duncan Hines)	1/12 cake	312	32	11
Fruitcake	1½ oz	165	38	7
Gingerbread	1/9 cake	175	21	4
Lemon (Pillsbury)	1/12 cake	220	37	9
Pound Cake (Sara Lee)	1/10 cake	130	48	7
Sponge cake, homemade	2½ oz	201	14	3
White Cake (Duncan Hines)	1/12 cake	333	27	10
Yellow Cake (Pillsbury)	1/12 cake	310	29	10

SNACK CAKES

Product	Portion	Calories	Percent Calories from Fat	Fat Grams
Big Wheels	1	170	48	9
Choco-diles	1	240	41	11
Crumb Cake (Hostess)	1	130	28	4
Cupcake, Chocolate (Hostess)	1	170	32	6
Cupcake, Orange (Hostess)	1	150	30	5
Dessert Cups (Little Debbie)	1	80	11	1
Ding Dongs	1	170	48	9
Fruit Loaf (Hostess)	1	400	20	9

Product	Portion	Calories	Percent Calories from Fat	Fat Grams
CAKE				
SNACK CAKES				
Ho-Hos	1	120	45	6
Hostess-O's	1	240	41	11
Snoball	1	136	26	4
Suzy Q, Banana	1	240	34	9
Suzy Q, Chocolate	1	240	38	10
Swiss Roll (Tastykake)	1	280	39	12
Tiger Tail	1	210	26	6
Twinkies	1	160	28	5
Yodel (Drake's)	1	115	39	5
CANDY				
Baby Ruth	1 bar	260	42	12
Butterfinger	1 bar	260	42	12
Butterscotch candy	1 oz	113	8	1
Caramels	1 oz	113	24	3
Charleston Chew	1 bar	240	23	6
Gum drops	1 oz	98	0	0
Hard candy	1 oz	109	0	0
Jelly beans	1 oz	104	0	0
Lifesavers	1	10	0	0
M&M's, Peanut	1 bag	240	49	13
M&M's, Plain	1 bag	240	38	10
Marshmallows	1	19	0	0
Milk Chocolate (Hershey)	1 bar	254	53	15
Milk Chocolate with Almonds (Hershey)	1 bar	246	55	15

Product	Portion	Calories	Percent Calories from Fat	Fat Grams
CANDY				
Milky Way	1 bar	290	34	11
Mr. Goodbar	1 bar	296	58	19
Peanut Bar (Planters)	1 bar	240	53	14
Reese's Peanut Butter Cups	2	280	23	7
Skor	1 bar	220	57	14
Snickers	1 bar	290	43	14
Thin Mint (Nabisco)	1	42	21	1
Toffee (Kraft)	1 pc	30	30	1
CEREALS				
COLD CEREALS				
All-Bran (Kellogg)	1 oz	70	6	<1
All-Bran with extra fiber (Kellogg)	1 oz	60	2	1
Alpha-Bits	1 oz	110	6	<1
Apple Jacks	1 oz	110	1	Tr
Bran Buds	1 oz	73	9	<1
Bran Chex	1 oz	90	7	<1
Bran Flakes	1 oz	90	0	0
Cap'n Crunch	1 oz	120	19	<3
Cap'n Crunch's Crunchberries	1 oz	120	20	<3
Cheerios	1 oz	110	15	2
Cocoa Crispies	1 oz	110	3	<1
Cocoa Pebbles	1 oz	110	9	1
Cocoa Puffs	1 oz	110	8	1
Cookie Crisp	1 oz	110	8	1
Corn Bran	1 oz	110	7	1
Corn Chex	1 oz	110	2	Tr

Product	Portion	Calories	Percent Calories from Fat	Fat Grams

CEREALS

COLD CEREALS

Product	Portion	Calories	Percent Calories from Fat	Fat Grams
Corn Flakes	1 oz	110	8	1
Corn Pops	1 oz	110	0	0
Cracklin' Oat Bran	1 oz	110	33	4
Crispix	1 oz	110	0	0
Crispy Wheats 'n Raisins	1 oz	110	4	<1
C. W. Post	1 oz	126	29	4
Fiber One	1 oz	60	15	1
Froot Loops	1 oz	110	4	<1
Frosted Flakes	1 oz	110	0	0
Frosted Mini-Wheats	1 oz	110	0	0
Fruit & Fiber	1 oz	90	10	1
Fruity Pebbles	1 oz	112	8	1
Golden Grahams	1 oz	110	8	1
Granola	1 oz	127	28	4
Grape-Nuts	1 oz	104	1	Tr
Grape-Nuts Flakes	1 oz	104	1	Tr
Heartland	1 oz	112	1	Tr
Honey Nut Cheerios	1 oz	110	8	1
Honey Smacks	1 oz	110	8	1
Honeycomb	1 oz	110	2	Tr
Kellogg's Corn Flakes	1 oz	110	8	1
Kellogg's Raisin Bran	1 oz	120	8	<1
Kix	1 oz	110	8	1
Life	1 oz	110	16	2
Lucky Charms	1 oz	110	8	1

Product	Portion	Calories	Percent Calories from Fat	Fat Grams

CEREALS

COLD CEREALS

Product	Portion	Calories	Percent Calories from Fat	Fat Grams
Nabisco Shredded Wheat	1 biscuit	84	1	Tr
Nabisco 100% Bran	1 oz	110	16	2
Nature Valley Granola	1 oz	126	36	5
Nutri-Grain, Corn	1 oz	110	8	1
Nutri-Grain, Rye	1 oz	102	2	Tr
Nutri-Grain, Wheat	1 oz	102	2	Tr
Pac-Man	1 oz	110	2	Tr
Post Raisin Bran	1 oz	90	4	<1
Post Toasties Corn Flakes	1 oz	110	2	<1
Product 19	1 oz	100	0	0
Puffed Rice	1 oz	55	2	Tr
Quaker 100% Natural Cereal	1 oz	136	37	6
Rice Chex	1 oz	110	2	<1
Rice Krispies	1 oz	110	0	0
Seven Grain	1 oz	110	8	1
Shredded Wheat 'n Bran	1 oz	110	8	1
Special K	1 oz	110	0	0
Sugar Frosted Flakes	1 oz	108	8	Tr
Sugar Golden Crisp	1 oz	104	1	Tr
Sugar Smacks	1 oz	106	4	<1
Total	1 oz	110	8	1

Product	Portion	Calories	Percent Calories from Fat	Fat Grams

CEREALS

COLD CEREALS
Trix	1 oz	110	8	1
Wheat Chex	1 oz	100	6	< 1
Wheaties	1 oz	100	5	< 1

HOT CEREALS
Bulgur	½ cup	113	4	< 1
Cream of Rice	½ cup	63	0	0
Cream of Wheat, quick	½ cup	73	3	Tr
Farina	½ cup	67	1	Tr
Hominy grits	½ cup	86	1	Tr
Malt-O-Meal	½ cup	61	1	Tr
Maypo	½ cup	85	13	1
Oatmeal (Quaker Old-Fashioned)	½ cup	105	15	< 2

CHEESE

NATURAL
Blue (Kraft)	1 oz	100	81	9
Brick	1 oz	105	69	8
Brie	1 oz	95	76	8
Burger Cheese (Sargento)	1 oz	106	76	9
Cajun (Sargento)	1 oz	110	74	9
Camembert	1 oz	85	74	7
Caraway	1 oz	100	72	8
Cheddar (Alpine Lace)	1 oz	97	74	8
Cheddar (Kraft)	1 oz	110	74	9

Product	Portion	Calories	Percent Calories from Fat	Fat Grams

CHEESE

NATURAL
Product	Portion	Calories	Percent Calories from Fat	Fat Grams
Cheddar, grated	1 cup	455	75	38
Cheshire	1 oz	110	74	9
Colby	1 oz	110	74	9
Colby-Jack (Sargento)	1 oz	109	74	9
Cottage, creamed	½ cup	117	38	5
Cottage, dry curd	½ cup	62	9	< 1
Cottage, 1% fat	½ cup	82	11	1
Cream Cheese	1 oz	99	91	10
Cream Cheese, light (Philadelphia)	1 oz	62	73	5
Edam	1 oz	100	72	8
Farmer's Cheese (White Clover)	1 oz	90	70	7
Feta	1 oz	90	70	7
Fontina	1 oz	110	74	9
Gorgonzola (Sargento)	1 oz	100	72	8
Gouda (Holland Farm)	1 oz	103	70	8
Gruyere	1 oz	117	69	9
Havarti (Casino)	1 oz	120	83	11
Jarlsberg	1 oz	100	63	7
Limburger	1 oz	93	77	8
Monterey Jack (Alpine Lace)	1 oz	80	45	4
Monterey Jack (Land O' Lakes)	1 oz	110	82	9

Product	Portion	Calories	Percent Calories from Fat	Fat Grams
CHEESE				
NATURAL				
Mozzarella, part skim (Polly-O)	1 oz	80	56	5
Mozzarella, whole milk (Polly-O)	1 oz	90	60	6
Mozzarella with Pizza Spices (Polly-O)	1 oz	79	57	5
Muenster	1 oz	110	74	9
Neufchatel	1 oz	74	62	7
Parmesan, grated	1 oz	130	62	9
Parmesan, hard	1 oz	111	57	7
Parmesan & Romano Grated Blend (Sargento)	1 oz	111	57	7
Port du Salut	1 oz	100	72	8
Provolone	1 oz	100	63	7
Queso Blanco (Sargento)	1 oz	104	78	9
Queso de Papa (Sargento)	1 oz	114	71	9
Ricotta, part skim (Polly-O)	1 oz	45	60	3
Ricotta, whole milk (Polly-O)	1 oz	50	100	7
Romano, grated (Polly-O)	1 oz	130	69	10
Roquefort	1 oz	105	77	9
String cheese	1 oz	79	57	5

Product	Portion	Calories	Percent Calories from Fat	Fat Grams

CHEESE

NATURAL

String cheese,
smoked	1 oz	79	57	5
Swiss	1 oz	110	65	8
Tilsit	1 oz	96	69	7

CHEESE FOOD

| American | 1 oz | 93 | 68 | 7 |

American
| (Hoffman's) | 1 oz | 100 | 63 | 7 |
| American (Kraft) | 1 oz | 90 | 70 | 7 |

American
| (Land O' Lakes) | 1 oz | 110 | 74 | 9 |

American,
| Imitation (Kraft) | 1 oz | 90 | 70 | 7 |

American Flavored
| (Light n' Lively) | 1 oz | 70 | 90 | 4 |

American Flavored
| (Light-Line) | 1 oz | 50 | 36 | 2 |

American Hot
Pepper
| (Sargento) | 1 oz | 106 | 76 | 9 |

American Spread
| (Sargento) | 1 oz | 106 | 76 | 9 |

American with
Pimento
| (Sargento) | 1 oz | 106 | 76 | 9 |

Babybel
(Fromageries
| Bel) | 1 oz | 91 | 69 | 7 |

Bombino
(Fromageries
| Bel) | 1 oz | 103 | 79 | 9 |

Product	Portion	Calories	Percent Calories from Fat	Fat Grams

CHEESE

CHEESE FOOD
Product	Portion	Calories	Percent Calories from Fat	Fat Grams
Bonbel (Fromageries Bel)	1 oz	100	72	8
Brick (Sargento)	1 oz	95	85	9
Cheddar (Cracker Barrel)	1 oz	90	70	7
Cheddar, Imitation (Sargento)	1 oz	85	64	6
Cheddar, Sharp (Hoffman's)	1 oz	110	65	8
Cheddar, Sharp (Wispride)	1 oz	100	63	7
Cheddar Flavored (Light n' Lively)	1 oz	70	51	4
Cheese Whiz	1 oz	80	68	6
Colby (Armour)	1 oz	110	74	9
Gruyere (Laughing Cow)	1 oz	72	75	6
Hickory Smoked (Wispride)	1 oz	100	54	7
Hot Pepper (Sargento)	1 oz	106	76	9
Italian Style Grated Cheese (Formagg)	1 oz	70	64	5
Jalapeno (Land O' Lakes)	1 oz	90	70	7
Limburger Spread (Mohawk Valley)	1 oz	70	77	6

Product	Portion	Calories	Percent Calories from Fat	Fat Grams
CHEESE				
CHEESE FOOD				
Monterey Jack (Armour)	1 oz	110	74	9
Monterey Jack (May-Bud)	1 oz	110	74	9
Monterey Jack (Kraft)	1 oz	90	70	7
Mozzarella (Formagg)	1 oz	70	64	5
Mozzarella, Imitation (Sargento)	1 oz	80	68	6
Onion (Land O' Lakes)	1 oz	90	70	7
Pimiento	1 oz	106	76	9
Port Wine Cheese Food (Wispride)	1 oz	100	63	7
Provolone (Formagg)	1 oz	70	64	5
Salami Cheese Food (Land O' Lakes)	1 oz	100	72	8
Smokey Sharp (Hoffman's)	1 oz	110	74	9
Spread (Golden Velvet)	1 oz	80	68	6
Swiss (Kraft)	1 oz	90	70	7
Swiss (Sargento)	1 oz	95	66	7
Swiss Flavor (Light n' Lively)	1 oz	70	51	4
Velveeta	1 oz	80	68	6

Product	Portion	Calories	Percent Calories from Fat	Fat Grams
CHEESE				
CHEESE SAUCE				
Canned				
(Campbell's)	2 oz	60	60	4
Dry mix	¼ cup	79	46	4
Land O' Lakes	2 oz	80	68	6
CHICKEN				
BROILERS AND FRYERS				
With skin, raw	3½ oz	215	3	15
With skin, batter dipped & fried	3½ oz	289	53	17
With skin, flour coated & fried	3½ oz	269	50	15
With skin, roasted	3½ oz	239	53	14
With skin, stewed	3½ oz	219	53	13
Flesh only, raw	3½ oz	119	23	3
Flesh only, fried	3½ oz	219	37	9
Flesh only, roasted	3½ oz	190	33	7
Flesh only, stewed	3½ oz	177	36	7
Skin only, batter dipped & fried	3½ oz	394	66	29
Skin only, flour coated & fried	3½ oz	502	75	42
Dark meat only, raw	3½ oz	125	29	4
Dark meat with skin, raw	3½ oz	237	68	18
Dark meat only, fried	3½ oz	239	45	12

Product	Portion	Calories	Percent Calories from Fat	Fat Grams

CHICKEN

BROILERS AND FRYERS

Product	Portion	Calories	Percent Calories from Fat	Fat Grams
Dark meat with skin, batter dipped & fried	3½ oz	298	54	18
Dark meat with skin, flour coated & fried	3½ oz	285	54	17
Dark meat only, roasted	3½ oz	205	44	10
Dark meat with skin, roasted	3½ oz	256	56	16
Dark meat only, stewed	3½ oz	192	28	6
Dark meat with skin, stewed	3½ oz	233	58	15
Light meat only, raw	3½ oz	114	8	1
Light meat with skin, raw	3½ oz	186	53	11
Light meat only, fried	3½ oz	192	42	9
Light meat with skin, batter dipped & fried	3½ oz	277	42	13
Light meat with skin, flour coated & fried	3½ oz	246	44	12
Light meat only, roasted	3½ oz	173	23	5
Light meat with skin, roasted	3½ oz	222	45	11

Product	Portion	Calories	Percent Calories from Fat	Fat Grams
CHICKEN				
BROILERS AND FRYERS				
Light meat only, stewed	3½ oz	159	23	4
Light meat with skin, stewed	3½ oz	201	45	10
CAPONS				
Meat with skin, raw	3½ oz	234	38	10
Meat with skin, roasted	3½ oz	229	47	12
PARTS				
Breast, meat only, raw	½ breast	129	7	1
Breast, meat with skin, raw	½ breast	250	47	13
Breast, meat only, fried	½ breast	161	22	4
Breast, meat with skin, batter dipped & fried	½ breast	364	45	18
Breast, meat with skin, flour coated & fried	½ breast	218	37	9
Breast, meat only, roasted	½ breast	142	19	3
Breast, meat with skin, roasted	½ breast	193	37	8
Drumstick, meat only, raw	1 drumstick	74	24	2
Drumstick, meat with skin, raw	1 drumstick	117	46	6

Product	Portion	Calories	Percent Calories from Fat	Fat Grams
CHICKEN				
PARTS				
Drumstick, meat only, fried	1 drumstick	82	33	3
Drumstick, meat with skin, batter dipped & fried	1 drumstick	193	51	11
Drumstick, meat with skin, flour coated & fried	1 drumstick	120	53	7
Drumstick, meat only, roasted	1 drumstick	76	24	2
Drumstick, meat with skin, roasted	1 drumstick	112	48	6
Drumstick, meat only, stewed	1 drumstick	78	35	3
Drumstick, meat with skin, stewed	1 drumstick	116	47	6
Giblets, flour coated & fried	½ cup	201	45	10
Giblets, simmered	½ cup	114	14	4
Liver pâté	2 oz	114	63	8
Liver, simmered	3½ oz	157	34	6
Neck, fried	1 neck	119	68	9
Neck, simmered	1 neck	94	67	7
Thigh, meat only, raw	1 thigh	82	33	3
Thigh, meat with skin, raw	1 thigh	199	63	14
Thigh, meat only, fried	1 thigh	113	40	5

Product	Portion	Calories	Percent Calories from Fat	Fat Grams

CHICKEN

PARTS

Product	Portion	Calories	Percent Calories from Fat	Fat Grams
Thigh, meat with skin, batter dipped & fried	1 thigh	238	53	14
Thigh, meat with skin, flour coated & fried	1 thigh	162	50	9
Thigh, meat only, roasted	1 thigh	109	50	6
Thigh, meat with skin, roasted	1 thigh	153	59	10
Thigh, meat only, stewed	1 thigh	107	42	5
Thigh, meat with skin, stewed	1 thigh	158	57	10
Wing, meat only	1 wing	36	25	1
Wing, meat with skin, raw	1 wing	109	66	8
Wing, meat only, fried	1 wing	42	43	2
Wing, meat with skin, batter dipped & fried	1 wing	159	62	11
Wing, meat with skin, flour coated & fried	1 wing	103	61	7
Wing, meat only, roasted	1 wing	43	42	2
Wing, meat with skin, roasted	1 wing	99	64	7
Wing, meat only, stewed	1 wing	43	42	2

Product	Portion	Calories	Percent Calories from Fat	Fat Grams

CHICKEN

PARTS
Wing, meat with
  skin, stewed | 1 wing | 100 | 63 | 7

ROASTERS
Meat with skin,
  roasted | 3½ oz | 223 | 52 | 13
Meat only, roasted | 3½ oz | 223 | 52 | 13
Dark meat only,
  roasted | 3½ oz | 178 | 46 | 9
Light meat only,
  roasted | 3½ oz | 153 | 24 | 4

CHICKEN PRODUCTS
Batter Gold
  (Tyson) | 3½ oz | 285 | 60 | 19
Breast Strips
  (Tyson) | 3½ oz | 270 | 43 | 13
Buttermilk (Tyson) | 3½ oz | 285 | 63 | 20
Cutlet, breaded
  and fried
  (Perdue) | 1 cutlet | 240 | 41 | 11
Delecta Delicious
  (Tyson) | 3½ oz | 305 | 56 | 19
Heat n' Serve
  (Tyson) | 3½ oz | 270 | 57 | 17
Honey Stung
  (Tyson) | 3½ oz | 260 | 48 | 14
Lightly Breaded
  (Tyson) | 3½ oz | 255 | 49 | 14

Product	Portion	Calories	Percent Calories from Fat	Fat Grams
CHICKEN				
CHICKEN PRODUCTS				
Liver Pâté	2 oz	114	63	8
Nuggets, breaded and fried (Perdue)	4 nuggets	240	41	11
Roll, light meat (Perdue)	3½ oz	159	40	7
Sandwich Mate (Tyson)	3½ oz	315	57	20
School Lunch Patty (Tyson)	3½ oz	290	62	20
Tenders, breaded and fried (Perdue)	3½ oz	185	54	11
CHOCOLATE				
Chips (Baker's)	¼ cup	196	41	9
Chips, semisweet (Baker's)	¼ cup	202	53	12
Chips, semisweet (Hershey)	¼ cup	228	51	13
Semi-Sweet (Baker's)	1 oz	136	60	9
Sweetened (Hershey)	1 oz	150	48	8
Unsweetened (Baker's)	1 oz	142	95	15
Unsweetened (Hershey)	1 oz	190	57	12

Product	Portion	Calories	Percent Calories from Fat	Fat Grams

CONDIMENTS

Product	Portion	Calories	Percent Calories from Fat	Fat Grams
A-1 Steak Sauce (Heublein)	1 tbsp	14	6	Tr
Au jus gravy, canned	¼ cup	10	9	Tr
Au jus gravy, mix, prepared with water	¼ cup	5	18	Tr
Barbecue sauce	¼ cup	47	19	1
Barbecue Sauce (Kraft)	1 tbsp	23	20	< 1
Barbecue Sauce, Hickory (Open Pit)	1 tbsp	23	20	< 1
Bearnaise sauce, dried, prepared with milk and butter	½ cup	350	10	34
Beef gravy, canned	¼ cup	31	29	1
Brown gravy, mix, prepared with water	¼ cup	3	0	0
Catsup	1 tbsp	16	6	Tr
Cheese sauce, dried, prepared with milk	¼ cup	77	50	4
Chicken gravy, canned	¼ cup	48	66	4
Chicken gravy, mix, prepared with water	¼ cup	21	21	< 1
Chili Sauce (Heinz)	1 tbsp	17	0	0
Curry sauce, mix, prepared with milk	¼ cup	68	50	4

Product	Portion	Calories	Percent Calories from Fat	Fat Grams

CONDIMENTS

Product	Portion	Calories	Percent Calories from Fat	Fat Grams
Hollandaise, mix, prepared with milk and butter	¼ cup	175	87	17
Horseradish	1 tbsp	6	0	0
Horseradish Sauce (Kraft)	1 tbsp	50	90	5
Mayonnaise (Best)	1 tbsp	100	99	11
Mayonnaisse (Hellman's)	1 tbsp	100	99	11
Mayonnaisse (Kraft)	1 tbsp	100	100	12
Mayonnaise, imitation	1 tbsp	15	60	1
Mayonnaise, imitation (Miracle Whip)	1 tbsp	70	90	7
Mayonnaise, reduced calorie	1 tbsp	40	90	4
Mushroom gravy, canned	¼ cup	30	45	<2
Mushroom gravy, mix, prepared with water	¼ cup	18	13	Tr
Mushroom sauce, dried, prepared with milk	¼ cup	127	23	3
Mustard (Grey Poupon)	1 tbsp	18	50	1
Mustard (Heinz)	1 tbsp	15	36	<1
Mustard, brown	1 tbsp	15	54	<1
Mustard, yellow	1 tbsp	12	45	<1

Product	Portion	Calories	Percent Calories from Fat	Fat Grams

CONDIMENTS

Product	Portion	Calories	Percent Calories from Fat	Fat Grams
Onion gravy, mix, prepared with water	¼ cup	20	11	Tr
Pesto (Fresh Chef)	¼ cup	315	86	30
Picante Sauce (Ortega)	¼ cup	20	0	0
Pork gravy, mix, prepared with water	¼ cup	19	24	< 1
Soy sauce	1 tbsp	11	8	Tr
Stroganoff sauce, dried, prepared with milk and water	¼ cup	73	37	3
Sweet and Sour Sauce (La Choy)	1 tbsp	30	3	Tr
Sweet and Sour Sauce (Kikkoman)	1 tbsp	18	5	Tr
Tabasco sauce	1 tbsp	Tr	0	0
Taco Salsa (Ortega)	1 tbsp	5	0	0
Taco Sauce (Ortega)	1 tbsp	6	0	0
Tartar Sauce (Best Foods)	1 tbsp	70	100	8
Tartar Sauce (Hellman's)	1 tbsp	70	100	8
Teriyaki sauce, bottled	1 tbsp	15	0	0
Teriyaki sauce, dried, prepared with water	1 tbsp	8	11	Tr

Product	Portion	Calories	Percent Calories from Fat	Fat Grams
CONDIMENTS				
Turkey gravy, canned	¼ cup	31	36	1
Turkey gravy, mix, prepared with water	¼ cup	22	20	<1
White sauce, mix	¼ cup	151	48	8
Worcestershire sauce	1 tbsp	59	2	Tr
COOKIES				
Animal (Barnum's)	6	70	18	<2
Apple Bars (Nabisco)	1	110	16	2
Apple Fruit Sticks (Almost Home)	1	70	26	2
Applesauce Raisin (Almost Home)	2	140	51	8
Arrowroot Biscuit (National)	6	130	28	4
Blueberry Newtons (Nabisco)	1	110	16	2
Brownie, homemade	1	95	57	6
Butter Flavored Cookies (Sunshine)	6	180	38	8
Creme Filled (Cameo)	2	140	32	5
Cherry Fruit Sticks (Almost Home)	1	70	26	2
Chocolate Chip (Duncan Hines)	2	144	44	7

Product	Portion	Calories	Percent Calories from Fat	Fat Grams
COOKIES				
Chocolate Chip (Chips Ahoy)	3	140	45	7
Chocolate Chip, from refrigerated dough (Pillsbury)	3	140	45	7
Chocolate Grahams (Nabisco)	3	150	42	7
Date Pecan (Pepperidge Farm)	3	170	42	8
Fig Newtons	2	100	18	2
Fudge Chocolate Chip (Almost Home)	2	130	35	5
Fudge 'n Chocolate Creme Sandwich (Almost Home)	2	280	39	12
Fudge Cremes (Keebler)	4	136	42	6
Gingersnaps, homemade	4	136	42	6
Gingersnaps (Nabisco)	4	120	23	3
Graham (Honey Maid)	4	120	15	2
Ladyfingers	4	158	19	3
Mallowmars	2	130	42	6
Mystic Mint	2	130	42	6
Oatmeal (Almost Home)	2	130	35	5

Product	Portion	Calories	Percent Calories from Fat	Fat Grams
COOKIES				
Oatmeal Raisin, from refrigerated dough (Pillsbury)	2	200	25	6
Oatmeal Raisin (Almost Home)	2	130	35	5
Oreos	3	140	39	6
Peanut Butter (Almost Home)	3	210	54	13
Peanut Butter, from refrigerated dough (Pillsbury)	3	200	38	8
Seville (Pepperidge Farm)	2	100	45	5
Shortbread (Lorna Doone)	4	140	45	7
Social Tea Biscuits (Nabisco)	6	130	28	4
Sugar, from refrigerated dough (Pillsbury)	3	201	36	8
Sugar Wafers (Sunshine)	3	130	42	6
Vanilla Wafers (Keebler)	3	60	45	3
CRACKERS				
Cheez-It (Sunshine)	6	35	51	2
Chicken in a Basket (Nabisco)	7	70	51	4

Product	Portion	Calories	Percent Calories from Fat	Fat Grams
CRACKERS				
Crispbread (Kavli)	2	30	3	Tr
Cracked Wheat (Pepperidge Farm)	4	110	33	4
Escort (Nabisco)	3	80	45	4
Matzoh	1	117	1	Tr
Melba toast	2	30	0	0
Ritz	9	150	48	8
Rye Wafer	2	45	4	< 1
Saltine	4	52	21	1
Sesame (Pepperidge Farm)	4	80	34	3
Soda	4	60	15	1
Stoned Wheat (FFV)	4	60	15	1
Tid-Bit Cheese (Nabisco)	8	35	51	2
Tiny Goldfish, Original (Pepperidge Farm)	10	35	51	2
Town House (Keebler)	9	157	52	9
Triscuit	3	60	30	2
Uneeda Biscuit	3	60	30	2
Waverley Crackers (Nabisco)	4	70	39	3
Wheat Thins (Nabisco)	4	35	39	2
Wheat Wafers (Sunshine)	4	40	45	2
Zwieback (Nabisco)	2	60	15	1

Product	Portion	Calories	Percent Calories from Fat	Fat Grams

DIET FOODS AND DRINKS

DIET BARS
Slender Chocolate	2	270	47	14
Slender Vanilla	2	270	50	15

DIET DRINKS
Chocolate Fudge Shake Mix (Weight Watchers)	12 fl oz	70	13	1
Fit & Frosty, Chocolate	8 fl oz	70	0	0
Fit & Frosty, Strawberry	8 fl oz	70	0	0
Fit & Frosty, Vanilla	8 fl oz	70	0	0
Orange Sherbet Shake Mix (Weight Watchers)	12 fl oz	70	0	0
Slender Chocolate Malt, canned	10 fl oz	220	16	4
Slender Strawberry Malt, canned	10 fl oz	220	16	4
Slender Vanilla Malt, canned	10 fl oz	220	16	4

DINNERS

ARMOUR CLASSIC LITE DINNERS
Baby Bay Shrimp	10½ oz	260	21	6
Beef Pepper Steak	10½ oz	260	21	6

Product	Portion	Calories	Percent Calories from Fat	Fat Grams

DINNERS

ARMOUR CLASSIC LITE DINNERS

Product	Portion	Calories	Percent Calories from Fat	Fat Grams
Chicken Breast Marsala	10½ oz	290	28	9
Chicken Burgundy	10 oz	210	9	2
Chicken Cacciatore	11 oz	250	14	4
Chicken Oriental	11 oz	250	14	4
Salisbury Steak	10 oz	270	43	13
Seafood with Natural Herbs	10½ oz	220	16	4
Steak Diane	10 oz	290	28	9
Sweet & Sour Chicken	10½ oz	240	8	2

ARMOUR DINNER CLASSICS

Product	Portion	Calories	Percent Calories from Fat	Fat Grams
Beef Burgundy	10 oz	460	65	33
Beef Stroganoff	10 oz	320	34	12
Boneless Beef Short Ribs	10½ oz	320	34	12
Chicken Fricassee	11¾ oz	340	29	12
Salisbury Steak	11 oz	460	49	25
Seafood Newburg	11½ oz	300	36	12
Sirloin Tips	11 oz	290	31	10
Swedish Meatballs	12½ oz	480	51	27
Veal Parmigiana	10¾ oz	400	50	22

BANQUET DINNERS

Product	Portion	Calories	Percent Calories from Fat	Fat Grams
Beans & Frankfurters	10 oz	510	44	25
Chopped Beef	11 oz	420	66	31
Meat Loaf	11 oz	440	55	27
Salisbury Steak	11 oz	495	62	34
Turkey	10½ oz	385	47	20

Product	Portion	Calories	Percent Calories from Fat	Fat Grams
DINNERS				
BANQUET DINNERS				
Western	11 oz	630	57	40
BANQUET EXTRA HELPING DINNERS				
Beef	16 oz	865	63	61
Lasagna	16½ oz	645	32	23
Salisbury Steak	18 oz	910	59	60
Salisbury Steak with Mushroom Gravy	18 oz	890	59	58
Turkey	19 oz	750	49	41
BANQUET FAMILY FAVORITE DINNERS				
Chicken & Dumplings	10 oz	420	51	24
Macaroni & Cheese	10 oz	415	43	20
Noodles & Chicken	10 oz	340	40	15
Spaghetti & Meatballs	10 oz	290	28	9
BANQUET PLATTERS				
Beef	10 oz	400	63	00
Chicken Nuggets	6½ oz	425	44	21
Fish	8¾ oz	445	44	22
Fried Chicken, white meat	9 oz	430	44	21
Ham	10 oz	400	36	16
MORTON DINNERS				
Beans & Franks	10 oz	360	35	14
Chicken Wings	6¾ oz	434	52	25
Fish & Chips	7¾ oz	386	35	15
Fried Chicken	7¾ oz	472	44	23

Product	Portion	Calories	Percent Calories from Fat	Fat Grams

DINNERS

MORTON DINNERS

Product	Portion	Calories	Percent Calories from Fat	Fat Grams
Salisbury Steak	7¾ oz	307	53	18
Sliced Beef	7¾ oz	248	29	8
Southern Fried Chicken Nuggets	6¾ oz	472	51	27
Turkey & Dressing	9 oz	216	17	4

NOODLE-RONI PASTA, FROM BOX MIX

Product	Portion	Calories	Percent Calories from Fat	Fat Grams
Chicken & Mushroom	8 oz	300	18	6
Fettucini	8 oz	600	51	34
Garlic & Butter	8 oz	580	50	32
Herbs & Butter	8 oz	320	39	14
Parmesano	8 oz	460	51	26
Pesto Italiano	8 oz	420	47	22
Rominoff	8 oz	480	41	22
Stroganoff	8 oz	480	49	26

SWANSON DINNERS

Product	Portion	Calories	Percent Calories from Fat	Fat Grams
Beans & Franks	10½ oz	420	36	17
Beef	11¼ oz	350	21	8
Chicken Nuggets	8¾ oz	470	48	25
Fish n' Fries	7¼ oz	420	45	21
Fried Chicken	10¾ oz	583	48	31
Macaroni & Cheese	12¼ oz	380	36	15
Meat Loaf	10¾ oz	430	44	21
Spaghetti & Meatballs	12½ oz	370	36	15
Turkey	8¾ oz	270	37	11

SWANSON HUNGRY MAN DINNERS

Product	Portion	Calories	Percent Calories from Fat	Fat Grams
Chicken Nuggets	16 oz	600	39	26
Chicken Parmigiana	20 oz	810	57	51

Product	Portion	Calories	Percent Calories from Fat	Fat Grams
DINNERS				
SWANSON HUNGRY MAN DINNERS				
Fish n' Chips	14¾ oz	780	45	39
Fried Chicken (Dark Meat)	11 oz	630	51	36
Fried Chicken (White Meat)	11¾ oz	680	50	38
Salisbury Steak	11¾ oz	610	56	38
Turkey	13¼ oz	390	32	14
Veal Parmigiana	18¼ oz	630	43	30
WEIGHT WATCHERS DINNERS				
Beef Stroganoff	9 oz	340	40	15
Cheese Manicotti	9¼ oz	300	39	13
Chicken a la King	9 oz	230	31	8
Chicken Parmigiana	8 oz	280	51	16
Filet of Fish	9¼ oz	210	26	6
Imperial Chicken	9¼ oz	230	16	4
Lasagna	11 oz	340	37	14
Oven Fried Fish	6¾ oz	220	49	12
Pasta Primavera	8½ oz	290	40	13
Southern Fried Chicken	6½ oz	270	53	16
Stuffed Sole with Newburg Sauce	10½ oz	310	26	9
Stuffed Turkey Breast	8½ oz	270	33	10
DIPS				
Acapulco	1 oz	8	0	0
Bacon & Horseradish	1 oz	60	75	5
Blue Cheese (Kraft)	1 oz	45	80	4

Product	Portion	Calories	Percent Calories from Fat	Fat Grams
DIPS				
Clam (Kraft)	1 oz	45	80	4
Creamy Cucumber (Kraft)	1 oz	45	80	4
Creamy Onion (Kraft)	1 oz	45	80	4
French Onion (Kraft)	1 oz	60	60	4
Garlic (Kraft)	1 oz	60	60	4
Green Onion (Kraft)	1 oz	60	60	4
Guacamole (Kraft)	1 oz	50	72	4
Jalapeno (Kraft)	1 oz	50	72	4
Jalapeno (Wise)	1 oz	25	0	0
Nacho Cheese (Kraft)	1 oz	50	72	4
Picante (Wise)	1 oz	12	0	0
Sour Cream, Flavored (Land O' Lakes)	1 oz	40	68	3
Taco (Wise)	1 oz	12	0	0
DUCK				
Flesh and skin, raw	3½ oz	404	89	40
Flesh only, roasted	3½ oz	201	49	11
Flesh and skin, roasted	3½ oz	337	75	28
EGGS				
CHICKEN EGGS				
Boiled	1 large	79	64	6
Fried	1 large	83	69	6
Omelet, plain	1 large	95	67	7
Poached	1 large	79	64	6

Product	Portion	Calories	Percent Calories from Fat	Fat Grams

EGGS

CHICKEN EGGS

Scrambled, with milk	1 large	95	67	7
White	1 large	16	0	0
Yolk	1 large	63	80	6

OTHER EGGS

Duck, whole	1	130	66	10
Goose, whole	1	276	62	19
Quail, whole	1	14	64	1
Turkey, whole	1	135	63	9

EGG SUBSTITUTES

Country Morning	¼ cup	87	62	6
Egg Beaters	¼ cup	25	0	0
Egg Beaters with Cheez	¼ cup	65	42	3
Egg Watchers (Tofutti)	¼ cup	50	36	2
Eggstra (Tillie Lewis)	¼ cup	43	2	1
Frozen	¼ cup	96	63	7
Powder	⅓ oz	44	27	1
Scrambled (Land O' Lakes)	¼ cup	72	100	9
Scramblers (Morningstar Farms)	¼ cup	58	31	2

ENTREES

GENERIC RECIPES

Beef and vegetable stew	1 cup	210	43	10

Product	Portion	Calories	Percent Calories from Fat	Fat Grams

ENTREES

GENERIC RECIPES

Product	Portion	Calories	Percent Calories from Fat	Fat Grams
Cheese soufflé	1 cup	308	73	25
Chicken a la king	1 cup	315	60	21
Chicken and noodles	1 cup	250	29	8
Chicken cacciatore	1 cup	525	55	32
Chicken chow mein	1 cup	255	35	10
Chicken pot pie	1 cup	510	58	33
Chili	1 cup	399	32	14
Chop suey with pork	1 cup	375	70	29
Crab, deviled	1 cup	364	59	24
Crab imperial	1 cup	323	45	16
Lasagna	1 cup	340	50	19
Lobster Newburg	1 cup	485	50	27
Macaroni and cheese	1 cup	430	48	23
Rigatoni with sausage sauce	1 cup	345	42	16
Spaghetti with meatballs	1 cup	332	33	12
Veal parmigiana	1 cup	550	59	36

CELENTANO FROZEN PASTA

Product	Portion	Calories	Percent Calories from Fat	Fat Grams
Canneloni Florentine	12 oz	380	40	17
Cavatelli	6½ oz	540	3	2
Cheese Ravioli	6½ oz	410	26	12
Chicken Parmigiana	9 oz	310	15	5
Chicken Primavera	11½ oz	270	30	9
Eggplant Parmigiana	8 oz	330	60	22

Product	Portion	Calories	Percent Calories from Fat	Fat Grams

ENTREES

CELENTANO FROZEN PASTA

Product	Portion	Calories	Percent Calories from Fat	Fat Grams
Lasagna	8 oz	320	45	16
Lasagna Primavera	11 oz	300	27	9
Manicotti with Sauce	8 oz	300	45	15
Stuffed Shells with Sauce	8 oz	320	39	14

CHUN KING DIVIDER PAK CANNED ENTREES

Product	Portion	Calories	Percent Calories from Fat	Fat Grams
Beef Chow Mein	7 oz	100	18	2
Beef Pepper Oriental	7 oz	110	33	4
Chicken Chow Mein	7 oz	110	33	4
Pork Chow Mein	7 oz	120	30	4
Shrimp Chow Mein	7 oz	100	18	2

CHUN KING STIR-FRY CANNED ENTREES

Product	Portion	Calories	Percent Calories from Fat	Fat Grams
Egg Foo Yung	5 oz	140	51	8
Chow Mein with Beef	6 oz	290	59	19
Chow Mein with Chicken	6 oz	220	45	11
Pepper Steak	6 oz	260	59	17

FRANCO-AMERICAN CANNED PASTA

Product	Portion	Calories	Percent Calories from Fat	Fat Grams
Beef Ravioli with Sauce	7½ oz	230	20	5
Macaroni and Cheese	7⅜ oz	170	26	5
Spaghetti with Sauce	7⅜ oz	190	9	2
Spaghetti-O's with Sauce	7⅜ oz	170	11	2

Product	Portion	Calories	Percent Calories from Fat	Fat Grams

ENTREES

FRANCO-AMERICAN CANNED PASTA

Product	Portion	Calories	Percent Calories from Fat	Fat Grams
Spaghetti and Meatballs with Sauce	7⅜ oz	220	33	8

LIPTON POUR-A-QUICHE

Product	Portion	Calories	Percent Calories from Fat	Fat Grams
3-Cheese	4⅓ oz	230	74	19
Bacon & Onion	4⅓ oz	230	70	18
Ham	4⅓ oz	230	67	17
Spinach & Onion	4⅓ oz	220	65	16

MRS. PAUL'S LIGHT SEAFOOD ENTREES

Product	Portion	Calories	Percent Calories from Fat	Fat Grams
Fish & Pasta Florentine	9½ oz	240	34	9
Fish au Gratin	10 oz	290	25	8
Fish Dijon	9½ oz	280	48	15
Fish Florentine	9 oz	210	17	4
Fish Mornay	10 oz	280	45	14
Shrimp & Clams with Linguini	10 oz	280	19	6
Shrimp Cajun Style	10½ oz	200	18	4
Shrimp Oriental	11 oz	280	16	5
Shrimp Primavera	11 oz	240	15	4
Tuna Pasta Casserole	11 oz	290	22	7

NOODLE-RONI PASTA, FROM BOX MIX

Product	Portion	Calories	Percent Calories from Fat	Fat Grams
Chicken & Mushroom	8 oz	300	18	6
Fettucine Alfredo	8 oz	600	51	34
Garlic & Butter	8 oz	580	50	32
Herbs & Butter	8 oz	320	39	14
Parmesano	8 oz	460	51	26
Pesto Italiano	8 oz	420	47	22

Product	Portion	Calories	Percent Calories from Fat	Fat Grams

ENTREES

NOODLE-RONI PASTA, FROM BOX MIX

Product	Portion	Calories	Percent Calories from Fat	Fat Grams
Rominoff	8 oz	480	41	22
Stroganoff	8 oz	480	49	26

STOUFFER'S ENTREES

Product	Portion	Calories	Percent Calories from Fat	Fat Grams
Beef Chop Suey with Rice	12 oz	300	27	9
Beef Pie	10 oz	500	58	32
Beef Stroganoff	9¾ oz	390	46	20
Cheese Enchiladas	10⅛ oz	590	61	40
Chicken Divan	8½ oz	320	56	20
Chicken Enchiladas	10 oz	490	53	29
Chicken Pie	10 oz	530	56	33
Ham & Asparagus Bake	9½ oz	510	62	35
Lasagna	10½ oz	360	83	13
Lobster Newburg	6½ oz	380	76	32
Macaroni & Beef	11½ oz	170	37	7
Macaroni & Cheese	12 oz	250	47	13
Salisbury Steak	9⅞ oz	250	50	14
Spaghetti with Meat Sauce	12⅞ oz	370	27	11
Tortellini, Beef with Marinara Sauce	10 oz	360	30	12
Tortellini, Cheese in Alfredo Sauce	8⅞ oz	600	60	40
Tortellini, Cheese with Tomato Sauce	9⅝ oz	360	40	16
Turkey Pie	10 oz	540	60	36

Product	Portion	Calories	Percent Calories from Fat	Fat Grams

ENTREES

STOUFFER'S ENTREES

Product	Portion	Calories	Percent Calories from Fat	Fat Grams
Vegetable Lasagna	10½ oz	420	51	24
STOUFFER'S LEAN CUISINE				
Beef & Pork Cannelloni with Mornay Sauce	9⅝ oz	260	35	10
Cheese Cannelloni	9⅛ oz	260	35	10
Chicken a l'Orange	8 oz	260	17	5
Chicken & Vegetables with Vermicelli	11¾ oz	270	27	8
Chicken Cacciatore with Vermicelli	10⅞ oz	250	25	7
Chicken Chow Mein	11¼ oz	250	18	5
Chicken Enchiladas	9⅞ oz	270	30	9
Chicken Marsala	8⅛ oz	190	24	5
Filet of Fish Divan	12⅜ oz	260	24	7
Filet of Fish Florentine	9 oz	240	34	9
Filet of Fish Jardiniere	11¼ oz	290	31	10
French Bread Pizza	5⅛ oz	310	26.	9
Glazed Chicken with Vegetable Rice	8½ oz	270	27	8
Linguine with Clam Sauce	9⅝ oz	270	23	7

Product	Portion	Calories	Percent Calories from Fat	Fat Grams
ENTREES				
STOUFFER'S LEAN CUISINE				
Meatball Stew	10 oz	250	36	10
Oriental Beef with Vegetables & Rice	8⅝ oz	250	25	7
Salisbury Steak	9½ oz	280	48	15
Shrimp & Chicken Cantonese	10⅛ oz	270	30	9
Spaghetti with Beef & Mushroom Sauce	11½ oz	280	23	7
Stuffed Cabbage	10¾ oz	220	41	10
Szechuan Beef with Noodles & Vegetables	9¼ oz	260	35	10
Tuna Lasagna	9¾ oz	270	33	10
Turkey Dijon	9½ oz	270	33	10
Vegetable & Pasta Mornay with Ham	9⅜ oz	280	35	11
Zucchini Lasagna	11 oz	260	24	7
STOUFFER'S RIGHT COURSE ENTREES				
Beef Dijon	9½ oz	290	28	9
Beef Ragout with Rice Pilaf	10 oz	300	24	9
Chicken Tenderloins in Barbecue Sauce	8¾ oz	270	20	6
Chicken Tenderloins in Peanut Sauce	9¼ oz	330	27	10

Product	Portion	Calories	Percent Calories from Fat	Fat Grams

ENTREES

STOUFFER'S RIGHT COURSE ENTREES

Product	Portion	Calories	Percent Calories from Fat	Fat Grams
Chicken Italiano	9⅝ oz	280	26	8
Fiesta Beef with Corn Pasta	8⅞ oz	270	23	7
Homestyle Pot Roast	9¼ oz	220	29	7
Sesame Chicken	10 oz	320	29	7
Sliced Turkey in a Mild Curry Sauce	8¾ oz	320	23	8
Shrimp Primavera	9⅝ oz	240	26	7
Vegetarian Chili	9¾ oz	280	23	7

SWANSON POT PIES

Product	Portion	Calories	Percent Calories from Fat	Fat Grams
Beef	10 oz	550	47	29
Chicken	10 oz	580	51	33
Turkey	10 oz	540	52	31

TYSON CHICKEN ENTREES

Product	Portion	Calories	Percent Calories from Fat	Fat Grams
Chicken Cordon Bleu	3½ oz	225	52	13
Chicken Kiev	3½ oz	290	68	22
Stuffed Chicken Breast	3½ oz	160	39	7

FAST FOOD

ARBY'S

Entrees

Product	Portion	Calories	Percent Calories from Fat	Fat Grams
Beef 'n Cheddar	1 sandwich	455	53	27
Chicken Breast	1 sandwich	493	46	25
Hot Ham 'n Cheese	1 sandwich	292	42	14

Product	Portion	Calories	Percent Calories from Fat	Fat Grams

FAST FOOD

ARBY'S
  Entrees
    Regular Roast

| Beef | 1 sandwich | 353 | 38 | 15 |
| Roast Chicken | 1 sandwich | 610 | 49 | 33 |

  Super Roast

| Beef | 1 sandwich | 501 | 40 | 22 |
| Turkey Deluxe | 1 sandwich | 375 | 40 | 17 |

Side Orders
  French Fries,

| regular | 1 order | 246 | 48 | 13 |
| Potato Cakes | 1 order | 204 | 53 | 12 |

Beverages

| Jamocha Shake | 11½ fl oz | 368 | 27 | 11 |

BURGER KING
  Entrees
    Bacon Double

| Cheeseburger | 1 | 515 | 54 | 31 |

Barbecue Bacon
  Double

| Cheeseburger | 1 | 536 | 52 | 31 |

BK Broiler
  Chicken

Sandwich	1	379	43	18
Cheeseburger	1	318	42	15
Chef Salad	1	178	46	9

Chicken

| Sandwich | 1 | 685 | 53 | 40 |
| Chicken Tenders | 6 pc | 236 | 50 | 13 |

Chunky Chicken

| Salad | 1 | 142 | 25 | 4 |

Product	Portion	Calories	Percent Calories from Fat	Fat Grams

FAST FOOD

BURGER KING
  Entrees
    Double
      Cheeseburger | 1 | 483 | 50 | 27
    Double Whopper | 1 | 935 | 59 | 61
    Fish Tenders | 6 pc | 267 | 54 | 16
    Hamburger | 1 | 272 | 36 | 11
    Ocean Catch
      Fish Filet | 1 | 495 | 45 | 25
    Mushroom Swiss
    Double
      Cheeseburger | 1 | 473 | 51 | 27
    Whopper | 1 | 614 | 53 | 36
    Whopper with
      Cheese | 1 | 706 | 56 | 44
  Side Orders
    French Fries,
      medium | 1 order | 341 | 53 | 20
    Garden Salad | 1 | 95 | 47 | 5
    Onion Rings | 1 order | 302 | 51 | 17
  Dessert
    Apple Pie | 4½ oz | 311 | 41 | 14
  Breakfast
    Bacon, Egg &
    Cheese
      Croissan'wich | 1 | 361 | 60 | 24
    Bagel Sandwich
    with Bacon,
      Egg & Cheese | 1 | 453 | 40 | 20
    Biscuit with
      Bacon & Egg | 1 | 467 | 52 | 27

Product	Portion	Calories	Percent Calories from Fat	Fat Grams
BURGER KING				
Entrees				
Double Cheeseburger	1	483	50	27
Double Whopper	1	935	59	61
Fish Tenders	6 pc	267	54	16
Hamburger	1	272	36	11
Ocean Catch Fish Filet	1	495	45	25
Mushroom Swiss Double Cheeseburger	1	473	51	27
Whopper	1	614	53	36
Whopper with Cheese	1	706	56	44
Side Orders				
French Fries, medium	1 order	341	53	20
Garden Salad	1	95	47	5
Onion Rings	1 order	302	51	17
Dessert				
Apple Pie	4½ oz	311	41	14
Breakfast				
Bacon, Egg & Cheese Croissan'wich	1	361	60	24
Bagel Sandwich with Bacon, Egg & Cheese	1	453	40	20
Biscuit with Bacon & Egg	1	467	52	27

Product	Portion	Calories	Percent Calories from Fat	Fat Grams

FAST FOOD

BURGER KING
Breakfast

Product	Portion	Calories	Percent Calories from Fat	Fat Grams
Biscuit with Sausage & Egg	1	568	57	36
French Toast Sticks	1 order	538	54	32
Hash Browns	1 order	213	51	12
Scrambled Egg Platter	1 order	549	56	34
Scrambled Egg Platter with Bacon	1 order	610	58	39

DAIRY QUEEN
Entrees

Product	Portion	Calories	Percent Calories from Fat	Fat Grams
Chicken Breast Fillet	1	608	50	34
Chicken Nuggets	1 order	276	59	18
Double Hamburger	1	530	48	28
Double Hamburger with Cheese	1	650	51	37
Fish Sandwich	1	430	38	18
Fish Sandwich with Cheese	1	483	41	22
Hamburger	1	360	40	16
Hamburger with Cheese	1	410	44	20
Super Hot Dog	1	520	47	27

Product	Portion	Calories	Percent Calories from Fat	Fat Grams

FAST FOOD

DAIRY QUEEN
  Entrees

Product	Portion	Calories	Percent Calories from Fat	Fat Grams
Super Hot Dog with Cheese	1	580	53	34
Super Hot Dog with Chili	1	570	51	32
Triple Hamburger	1	710	57	45
Triple Hamburger with Cheese	1	820	55	50

  Desserts

Product	Portion	Calories	Percent Calories from Fat	Fat Grams
Buster Bar	1	448	58	29
Chipper Sandwich	1	318	20	7
Chocolate Malt, regular	15 fl oz	760	21	18
Chocolate Shake, regular	15 fl oz	710	24	19
Chocolate Sundae, regular	6 oz	310	23	8
Dilly Bar	1	210	56	13
Dipped Chocolate Cone, regular	5½ oz	340	42	16
Float	14 fl oz	410	15	7
Freeze	14 fl oz	500	22	12
Fudge Nut Bar	1	406	55	25

Product	Portion	Calories	Percent Calories from Fat	Fat Grams

FAST FOOD

DAIRY QUEEN
Desserts

Product	Portion	Calories	Percent Calories from Fat	Fat Grams
Mr. Misty, regular	12 fl oz	250	0	0
Parfait	10 oz	430	17	8
Soft Ice Cream Cone, regular	5 oz	240	26	7
Vanilla Frozen Yogurt	4 oz	100	0	0

DOMINO'S PIZZA

Product	Portion	Calories	Percent Calories from Fat	Fat Grams
Cheese	2 slices	376	24	10
Deluxe	2 slices	498	37	20
Pepperoni	2 slices	460	35	18
Sausage	2 slices	430	33	16
Veggie	2 slices	498	33	19

JACK IN THE BOX
Entrees

Product	Portion	Calories	Percent Calories from Fat	Fat Grams
Bacon Cheeseburger	1	705	50	39
Cheeseburger	1	315	40	14
Chef Salad	1	325	50	18
Chicken Fajita Pita	1	292	25	8
Chicken Supreme	1	575	56	36
Double Cheeseburger	1	467	52	27
Fish Supreme	1	554	52	32

Product	Portion	Calories	Percent Calories from Fat	Fat Grams
FAST FOOD				
JACK IN THE BOX				
Entrees				
Grilled Chicken Fillet	1	408	38	17
Grilled Sourdough Burger	1	712	63	50
Ham & Turkey Melt	1	592	55	36
Hamburger	1	267	37	11
Jumbo Jack	1	584	52	34
Jumbo Jack with Cheese	1	677	53	40
Sirloin Cheesesteak	1	621	43	30
Swiss & Bacon Burger	1	678	62	47
Taco Salad	1	503	55	31
Side Orders				
French Fries, regular	1 order	353	48	19
Onion Rings	1 order	382	54	23
Beverages				
Chocolate Shake	11 fl oz	330	19	7
Strawberry Shake	11 fl oz	320	20	7
Vanilla Shake	11 fl oz	320	17	6
Breakfast				
Apple Turnover	1	410	53	24
Breakfast Jack	1	307	38	13

	Product	Portion	Calories	Percent Calories from Fat	Fat Grams

FAST FOOD

JACK IN THE BOX

Breakfast

Product	Portion	Calories	Percent Calories from Fat	Fat Grams
Pancake Platter	1	612	32	22
Sausage Crescent	1	584	66	43
Scrambled Egg Platter	1	662	54	40
Scrambled Egg Pocket	1	431	44	21
Supreme Crescent	1	547	66	40

KENTUCKY FRIED CHICKEN

Entrees

Product	Portion	Calories	Percent Calories from Fat	Fat Grams
Chicken Sandwich	1	482	50	27
Chicken Littles Sandwich	1	169	54	10
Extra Crispy Drumstick	1	204	61	14
Extra Crispy Center Breast	1	342	52	20
Extra Crispy Side Breast	1	343	59	22
Extra Crispy Thigh	1	406	66	30
Extra Crispy Wing	1	254	66	19
Hot Wings	6 pc	376	58	24
Kentucky Nuggets	6 pc	276	57	17

Product	Portion	Calories	Percent Calories from Fat	Fat Grams

FAST FOOD
KENTUCKY FRIED CHICKEN
Entrees

Product	Portion	Calories	Percent Calories from Fat	Fat Grams
Original Recipe Drumstick	1	146	52	9
Original Recipe Center Breast	1	283	49	15
Original Recipe Side Breast	1	267	56	17
Original Recipe Thigh	1	294	60	20
Original Recipe Wing	1	178	59	12
Side Orders				
Biscuit	1	235	45	12
Cole Slaw	1 order	119	50	7
Corn on the Cob	1 order	176	16	3
French Fries, regular	1 order	244	44	12
Mashed Potatoes & Gravy	1 order	71	20	<2

LONG JOHN SILVER'S
Entrees

Product	Portion	Calories	Percent Calories from Fat	Fat Grams
Batter-Fried Fish	1 pc	150	48	8
Batter-Fried Shrimp	1 pc	40	68	3
Batter-Fried Shrimp Dinner	6 pc	740	45	37
Breaded Clams	1 order	240	45	12
Breaded Shrimp	1 order	190	47	10

Product	Portion	Calories	Percent Calories from Fat	Fat Grams

FAST FOOD

LONG JOHN SILVER'S
  Entrees

Product	Portion	Calories	Percent Calories from Fat	Fat Grams
Breaded Shrimp Feast	13 pc	880	42	41
Catfish Fillet Dinner	2 fillets	860	44	42
Chicken Plank Dinner	4 pc	940	42	44
Clam Dinner	1 order	980	41	45
Fish & Chicken	1 order	870	41	40
Fish & Fries	2 pc	660	41	30
Fish & More	1 order	800	42	37
Fish Dinner	3 pc	960	41	44
Fish Sandwich Platter	1 order	870	39	38
Homestyle Fish	1 pc	125	50	7
Homestyle Fish Dinner	3 pc	880	43	42
Ocean Chef Salad	1 order	250	32	9
Seafood Platter	1 order	970	43	16
Seafood Salad	1 scoop	210	21	5
Shrimp & Fish Dinner	1 order	770	43	37
Shrimp, Fish & Chicken Dinner	1 order	840	43	40
Side Orders				
Clam Chowder	1 bowl	140	39	6
Cole Slaw	1 order	140	39	6

Product	Portion	Calories	Percent Calories from Fat	Fat Grams

FAST FOOD

LONG JOHN SILVER'S
  Side Orders
  Corn on the Cob

Product	Portion	Calories	Percent Calories from Fat	Fat Grams
with Whirl	1 order	270	47	14
French Fries	1 order	220	41	10
Gumbo	1 bowl	120	60	8
Hushpuppies	2 pc	140	26	4
Mixed Vegetables	1 order	60	30	2

  Dessert
  Lemon

Product	Portion	Calories	Percent Calories from Fat	Fat Grams
Meringue Pie	4 oz	260	24	7
Pecan Pie	4 oz	530	42	25

McDONALD'S
  Entrees

Product	Portion	Calories	Percent Calories from Fat	Fat Grams
Big Mac	1	560	52	32
Cheeseburger	1	310	40	14
Chef Salad	1 order	230	52	13
Chicken McNuggets	6 pc	290	51	16
Chicken Salad	1 order	140	22	3
Filet-O-Fish Sandwich	1	440	53	26
Hamburger	1	260	33	10
McChicken Sandwich	1	490	68	37
McD.L.T.	1 burger	580	57	37
McLean Deluxe	1 burger	320	28	10
Quarter Pounder	1	410	45	21
Quarter Pounder with Cheese	1	520	51	29

Product	Portion	Calories	Percent Calories from Fat	Fat Grams

FAST FOOD

McDONALD'S
Side Orders

Product	Portion	Calories	Percent Calories from Fat	Fat Grams
French Fries, medium	1 order	320	48	17
Garden Salad	1 order	110	54	7

Beverages

Product	Portion	Calories	Percent Calories from Fat	Fat Grams
Chocolate Shake	10¾ fl oz	390	24	11
Strawberry Shake	10¾ fl oz	380	24	10
Vanilla Shake	10¾ fl oz	350	26	10

Desserts

Product	Portion	Calories	Percent Calories from Fat	Fat Grams
Apple Pie	3 oz	260	51	15
Caramel Sundae	6¼ oz	340	24	9
Chocolaty Chip Cookies	1 box	330	43	16
Hot Fudge Sundae	1	310	27	9
McDonaldland Cookies	1 box	290	29	9
Soft Serve Cone	3 oz	140	29	5
Strawberry Sundae	6 oz	280	23	7

Breakfast

Product	Portion	Calories	Percent Calories from Fat	Fat Grams
Apple Danish	1	390	41	13
Biscuit with Bacon, Egg & Cheese	1	440	54	26
Biscuit with Sausage	1	440	59	29

Product	Portion	Calories	Percent Calories from Fat	Fat Grams

FAST FOOD

McDONALD'S
Breakfast

Product	Portion	Calories	Percent Calories from Fat	Fat Grams
Biscuit with Sausage & Egg	1	520	60	35
Cinnamon Raisin Danish	1	440	27	13
Egg McMuffin	1	290	35	11
English Muffin with Butter	1	170	24	5
Hash Browns	1 order	130	51	7
Hotcakes with Syrup & Butter	1 order	410	20	9
Sausage McMuffin	1	370	53	22
Sausage McMuffin with Egg	1	440	55	27
Scrambled Eggs	1 order	140	63	10

PIZZA HUT

Product	Portion	Calories	Percent Calories from Fat	Fat Grams
Hand-Tossed, Cheese	2 slices	518	35	20
Hand-Tossed, Pepperoni	2 slices	500	41	23
Hand-Tossed, Supreme	2 slices	540	43	26
Pan Pizza, Cheese	2 slices	492	33	18
Pan Pizza, Pepperoni	2 slices	540	37	22

2925
655
1270

Product	Portion	Calories	Percent Calories from Fat	Fat Grams

FAST FOOD

PIZZA HUT

Product	Portion	Calories	Percent Calories from Fat	Fat Grams
Pan Pizza, Supreme	2 slices	589	46	30
Personal Pan Pizza, Pepperoni	whole pizza	675	39	29
Personal Pan Pizza, Supreme	whole pizza	647	39	28
Thin 'n Crispy, Cheese	2 slices	398	38	17
Thin 'n Crispy, Pepperoni	2 slices	413	44	20
Thin 'n Crispy, Supreme	2 slices	459	43	22

ROY ROGERS

Entrees

Product	Portion	Calories	Percent Calories from Fat	Fat Grams
Bacon Cheeseburger	1	552	54	33
Cheeseburger	1	525	50	29
Chicken Breast	1	412	52	24
Chicken Leg	1	140	51	8
Chicken Nuggets	6 pc	288	56	18
Chicken Thigh	1	296	61	20
Chicken Wing	1	192	61	13
Fish Sandwich	1	514	42	24
Hamburger	1	472	55	29
Roast Beef Sandwich	1	350	28	11
Roast Beef Sandwich with Cheese	1	403	33	15

Product	Portion	Calories	Percent Calories from Fat	Fat Grams
FAST FOOD				
ROY ROGERS				
Entrees				
Roast Beef Sandwich, large	1	373	29	12
RR Bar Burger	1	573	49	31
Small Hamburger	1	222	36	9
Small Cheeseburger	1	275	43	13
Side Dishes				
Biscuit	1	231	47	12
Cole Slaw	1 order	110	57	7
French Fries, regular	1 order	320	45	16
Granola	¼ cup	65	42	3
Potato Salad	¼ cup	54	50	3
Beverages				
Chocolate Shake	1	358	25	10
Strawberry Shake	1	315	29	10
Vanilla Shake	1	306	32	11
Desserts				
Caramel Sundae	1	293	28	9
Hot Fudge Sundae	1	337	35	13
Strawberry Sundae	1	216	29	7

Product	Portion	Calories	Percent Calories from Fat	Fat Grams
FAST FOOD				
ROY ROGERS				
Breakfast				
Apple Swirls	1	328	19	7
Breakfast Crescent Sandwich	1	408	60	27
Breakfast Crescent Sandwich with Bacon	1	446	61	30
Breakfast Crescent Sandwich with Ham	1	456	57	29
Breakfast Crescent Sandwich with Sausage	1	564	67	42
Cheese Swirls	1	383	35	15
Egg & Biscuit Platter	1	557	55	34
Egg & Biscuit Platter with Bacon	1	607	58	39
Egg & Biscuit Platter with Ham	1	605	54	36
Egg & Biscuit Platter with Sausage	1	713	62	49

Product	Portion	Calories	Percent Calories from Fat	Fat Grams

FAST FOOD

ROY ROGERS
  Breakfast

Product	Portion	Calories	Percent Calories from Fat	Fat Grams
Pancake Platter	1	386	30	13
Pancake Platter with Bacon	1	436	35	17
Pancake Platter with Ham	1	434	31	15
Pancake Platter with Sausage	1	542	46	28

WENDY'S
  Entrees

Product	Portion	Calories	Percent Calories from Fat	Fat Grams
Bacon Cheeseburger	1	460	41	21
Cheeseburger	1	400	45	20
Chicken Sandwich	1	430	40	19
Chili	9 oz	220	29	7
Double Cheeseburger	1	640	54	38
Double Hamburger	1	570	52	33
Hamburger	1	340	40	15
Hamburger, Kid's Meal	1	260	31	9

  Side Dishes

Product	Portion	Calories	Percent Calories from Fat	Fat Grams
Baked Potato, plain	1	250	7	2
Baked Potato with Bacon & Cheese	1	450	36	18

Product	Portion	Calories	Percent Calories from Fat	Fat Grams

FAST FOOD

WENDY'S
  Side Dishes
    Baked Potato
      with Broccoli
      & Cheese

Baked Potato with Broccoli & Cheese	1	400	36	16
Baked Potato with Cheese	1	470	40	21
Baked Potato with Chili & Cheese	1	530	39	23
Baked Potato with Sour Cream & Chives	1	460	47	24
French Fries, regular	1 order	440	47	23
Pasta Salad	¼ cup	57	8	<1
Breakfast				
Breakfast Sandwich	1	370	46	19
French Toast	2 slices	400	43	19
Home Fries	1 order	360	55	22
Omelet #1, Ham & Cheese	1	290	65	21
Omelet #2, Ham, Cheese & Mushroom	1	250	61	17
Omelet #3, Ham, Cheese, Onion & Green Pepper	1	280	61	19

Product	Portion	Calories	Percent Calories from Fat	Fat Grams
FAST FOOD				
WENDY'S				
Breakfast				
Omelet #4, Mushroom, Onion & Green Pepper	1	210	64	15
Sausage	1 patty	200	81	18
Scrambled Eggs	1 order	190	57	12
FATS AND OILS				
Beef Tallow	1 tbsp	116	99	13
Butter	1 tbsp	108	100	12
Butter Blend (Blue Bonnet)	1 tbsp	90	100	11
Butter Blend (Country Morning)	1 tbsp	100	100	11
Chicken fat	1 tbsp	115	100	13
Goose fat	1 tbsp	115	100	13
I Can't Believe It's Not Butter (Lever)	1 tbsp	90	100	10
Lard	1 tbsp	115	100	13
Margarine, stick (Blue Bonnet)	1 tbsp	100	99	11
Margarine, stick (Fleishmann's)	1 tbsp	100	99	11
Margarine, stick (Land O' Lakes)	1 tbsp	100	99	11
Margarine, stick (Mazola)	1 tbsp	100	99	11
Margarine, squeeze (Fleishmann's)	1 tbsp	100	99	11

Product	Portion	Calories	Percent Calories from Fat	Fat Grams
FATS AND OILS				
Margarine, diet (Blue Bonnet)	1 tbsp	50	90	6
Margarine, diet (Mazola)	1 tbsp	50	90	6
Margarine, whipped (Blue Bonnet)	1 tbsp	70	89	7
Molly McButter	1 tbsp	24	0	0
Shortening (Crisco)	1 tbsp	106	100	12
Spread (Blue Bonnet)	1 tbsp	90	100	11
Spread, corn oil (Mazola)	1 tbsp	120	100	14
Spread, whipped (Blue Bonnet)	1 tbsp	70	89	7
Turkey fat	1 tbsp	115	100	13
Vegetable oil	1 tbsp	120	100	14
FISH				
Bass, striped, raw	3 oz	82	22	2
Bluefish, raw	3 oz	105	34	4
Caviar, sturgeon	1 tbsp	42	43	2
Chub, raw	3 oz	124	55	8
Clams, raw	6 large	95	9	1
Clam juice	3 fl oz	2	0	0
Cod, broiled	3 oz	89	10	1
Cod, dried, salted	3 oz	246	7	2
Cod, raw	3 oz	70	13	1
Crab, canned	3 oz	84	11	1
Crab, steamed	3 oz	82	11	1
Eel, broiled	3 oz	200	59	13
Fish fillets, frozen	3 oz	180	50	10
Fish sticks, frozen	3 sticks	228	39	10

Product	Portion	Calories	Percent Calories from Fat	Fat Grams
FISH				
Flatfish, raw	3 oz	78	12	1
Flounder, baked	3 oz	99	9	1
Frog legs, raw	3 oz	63	0	0
Haddock, broiled	3 oz	95	9	1
Haddock, raw	3 oz	74	12	1
Halibut, broiled	3 oz	119	15	2
Halibut, raw	3 oz	93	19	2
Herring, canned in oil	3 oz	192	52	11
Herring, raw	3 oz	134	54	8
Lobster, cooked	3 oz	83	11	1
Lobster, raw	3 oz	77	12	1
Mackerel, broiled	3 oz	223	61	15
Mackerel, canned	½ cup	148	36	6
Mackerel, raw	3 oz	174	62	12
MahiMahi, raw	3 oz	73	12	1
Oysters, raw	6 medium	58	31	2
Perch, raw	3 oz	80	11	1
SALMON				
Atlantic, raw	3 oz	121	37	5
Chinook, raw	3 oz	153	53	9
Chinook, smoked	3 oz	99	36	4
Coho, poached	3 oz	157	34	6
Coho, raw	3 oz	124	36	5
Sockeye (red), raw	3 oz	143	44	7
Sockeye (red), broiled	3 oz	183	44	9
Sardines in oil	3 oz	192	52	11
Scallops, fried	3 oz	201	46	10
Scallops, raw	3 oz	75	12	1
Shrimp, boiled	3 oz	84	11	1

Product	Portion	Calories	Percent Calories from Fat	Fat Grams
FISH				
Shrimp, fried	3 oz	206	44	10
Shrimp, raw	3 oz	90	10	1
Sole, raw	3 oz	58	4	Tr
Swordfish, broiled	3 oz	132	27	4
Trout, rainbow, broiled	3 oz	129	28	4
Trout, rainbow, raw	3 oz	100	27	3
TUNA				
Chunk Light in Oil (Bumble Bee)	3 oz	200	68	15
Chunk Light in Water (Bumble Bee)	3 oz	90	20	2
Chunk White in Oil (Bumble Bee)	3 oz	200	68	15
Chunk White in Water (Bumble Bee)	3 oz	90	20	2
Fresh, cooked	3 oz	157	29	5
Solid Light in Oil (Bumble Bee)	3 oz	190	47	10
Solid White in Water (Bumble Bee)	3 oz	90	20	2
FLOUR AND GRAINS				
All-Purpose Flour (Pillsbury Best)	1 cup	400	2	1
Barley flour	1 cup	401	4	2

Product	Portion	Calories	Percent Calories from Fat	Fat Grams
FLOUR AND GRAINS				
Barley, pearled, dry	1 cup	700	3	2
Bisquick (General Mills)	½ cup	480	30	16
Buckwheat flour	1 cup	340	3	1
Bulgur, cooked	1 cup	227	4	1
Corn bran	1 cup	165	8	< 2
Corn meal, degermed, cooked	1 cup	240	1	Tr
Cornmeal, degermed, dry	1 cup	138	13	2
Grits, cooked	1 cup	146	3	< 1
Oat bran	1 cup	270	20	6
Popcorn, popped	1 cup	30	8	Tr
Potato flour	1 cup	632	3	2
Rice, brown, cooked	1 cup	232	5	1
Rice, Chicken Flavored (Minute Rice)	1 cup	306	24	8
Rice, Drumstick Mix (Minute Rice)	1 cup	300	24	8
Rice, French Style (Birds Eye)	1 cup	220	1	Tr
Rice, Fried (Minute Rice)	1 cup	320	28	10
Rice, Long Grain & Wild (Minute Rice)	1 cup	300	24	8
Rice, Northern Italian Style (Birds Eye)	1 cup	240	8	2
Rice, Pilaf (Pritikin)	1 cup	180	1	Tr

Product	Portion	Calories	Percent Calories from Fat	Fat Grams

FLOUR AND GRAINS

Product	Portion	Calories	Percent Calories from Fat	Fat Grams
Rice, Rib Roast Mix (Minute Rice)	1 cup	300	24	8
Rice, Spanish (Pritikin)	1 cup	200	1	Tr
Rice, white, cooked	1 cup	223	1	Tr
Rice, white, dry	1 cup	670	13	1
Rice, wild, cooked	1 cup	296	24	8
Rice flour	1 cup	400	2	1
Rye flour, light	1 cup	364	2	1
Rye flour, dark	1 cup	419	7	3
Self-Rising Flour (Gold Medal)	1 cup	380	2	1
Soybean flour, defatted	1 cup	327	3	1
Wheat flour	1 cup	400	2	1
Wheat flour, cake	1 cup	430	2	1
Wheat germ, toasted	½ cup	216	25	6
White flour, all-purpose	1 cup	400	2	1
Whole wheat flour	1 cup	400	2	1

FRUIT

Product	Portion	Calories	Percent Calories from Fat	Fat Grams
Apple	1 large	57	4	Tr
Apple, canned, unsweetened	½ cup	69	13	1
Applesauce, unsweetened	½ cup	53	4	Tr
Apricots	2	32	7	Tr
Avocado	1	324	86	31
Banana	1	105	2	Tr

Product	Portion	Calories	Percent Calories from Fat	Fat Grams
FRUIT				
Blackberries	½ cup	37	7	Tr
Blueberries, canned	½ cup	118	2	Tr
Blueberries, frozen	½ cup	93	3	Tr
Boysenberries, canned	½ cup	113	2	Tr
Boysenberries, frozen	½ cup	33	5	Tr
Cantaloupe	1 cup	57	6	Tr
Cherries	10	49	13	< 1
Cherries, canned, unsweetened	½ cup	57	3	Tr
Cranberries	½ cup	23	4	Tr
Cranberry sauce, canned, sweetened	½ cup	209	1	Tr
Currants, red, raw	½ cup	31	3	Tr
Dates, dried	½ cup	230	0	0
Figs, dried	2	95	4	Tr
Fruit Salad (Kraft)	½ cup	50	0	0
Gooseberries	½ cup	34	12	Tr
Grapefruit	½ medium	39	2	Tr
Grapefruit, canned, unsweetened	½ cup	46	2	Tr
Grapes	½ cup	29	5	Tr
Grapes, canned	½ cup	94	1	Tr
Honeydew	½ cup	66	8	< 1
Mango	1 medium	135	4	< 1
Nectarine	1 medium	67	8	< 1
Orange	1 medium	65	1	Tr
Peach	1 medium	37	2	Tr
Peaches, cling, canned, unsweetened	½ cup	54	2	Tr

Product	Portion	Calories	Percent Calories from Fat	Fat Grams
FRUIT				
Pear	1 medium	98	9	1
Pears, canned, unsweetened	½ cup	35	3	Tr
Pineapple	½ cup	37	2	Tr
Pineapple, canned (Dole)	½ cup	95	1	Tr
Plum	1 medium	36	3	Tr
Prunes, dried	½ cup	113	1	Tr
Raisins	½ cup	225	0	Tr
Raspberries	½ cup	30	3	Tr
Rhubarb, cooked	½ cup	139	1	Tr
Strawberries	½ cup	23	4	Tr
Strawberries, frozen, unsweetened	½ cup	26	3	Tr
Tangerine	1 medium	37	2	Tr
Watermelon	½ cup	25	4	Tr
GOOSE				
Meat only, roasted	3 oz	204	49	11
Meat with skin, roasted	3 oz	261	66	19
Liver pâté	3 oz	393	85	37
HOT DOGS				
Beef	1	180	80	16
Beef (Armour)	1	170	79	15
Beef (Hebrew National)	1	160	84	15
Beef (Oscar Mayer)	1	144	81	13
Beef & Pork	1	144	81	13
Chicken	1	116	70	9

Product	Portion	Calories	Percent Calories from Fat	Fat Grams
HOT DOGS				
Chicken (Weaver)	1	115	78	10
Turkey	1	100	73	8
Turkey (Louis Rich)	1	103	74	9
Turkey with Cheese (Oscar Mayer)	1	103	73	8
ICE CREAM AND FROZEN DESSERTS				
Frozen yogurt, fruit	½ cup	108	8	1
Fruit 'n Juice Bar	1	75	6	< 1
Ice cream, chocolate	½ cup	264	44	13
Ice cream, strawberry	½ cup	226	40	10
Ice cream, vanilla	½ cup	135	47	7
Ice milk, vanilla	½ cup	92	33	3
Sherbet, orange	½ cup	135	13	2
Tofutti	½ cup	90	5	< 1
JAM, SUGAR, AND SYRUP				
Honey	1 tbsp	61	0	0
Jam, plum	1 tbsp	59	2	Tr
Jelly, strawberry	1 tbsp	51	0	0
Maple syrup	1 tbsp	50	0	0
Maple Syrup, Buttered (Log Cabin)	1 tbsp	105	9	1
Marmalade	1 tbsp	56	2	Tr
Sugar, white	1 tbsp	46	0	0
Sweet 'n Low	1 pkg	4	0	0

Product	Portion	Calories	Percent Calories from Fat	Fat Grams
LAMB				

Note: All figures are for separable lean only.

Product	Portion	Calories	Percent Calories from Fat	Fat Grams
Leg, roasted	3 oz	158	34	6
Loin chop, broiled	3 oz	180	40	8
Rib chop, roasted	3 oz	195	48	11
Shoulder, roasted	3 oz	174	44	9

MILK AND MILK BEVERAGES

Product	Portion	Calories	Percent Calories from Fat	Fat Grams
CREAM				
Half-and-half	½ cup	158	80	14
Heavy (whipping)	½ cup	411	96	44
Light	½ cup	235	88	23
Medium	½ cup	292	92	30
Nondairy Creamer (Coffee-Mate)	1 tsp	10	9	Tr
Nondairy Creamer (Coffee-Rich)	½ oz	22	82	2
Nondairy Creamer (Cremora)	1 tsp	12	75	1
Sour	½ cup	247	87	24
Sour, nondairy	½ cup	240	86	23
Whipped Topping (Kraft)	½ cup	70	77	6
Whipped topping, nondairy	½ cup	120	75	10
MILK				
Buttermilk, cultured	1 cup	99	18	2
Buttermilk, dry	1 tbsp	25	4	Tr
Condensed, sweetened	½ cup	492	26	14

Product	Portion	Calories	Percent Calories from Fat	Fat Grams

MILK AND MILK BEVERAGES

MILK
Evaporated, skim	½ cup	100	1	Tr
Evaporated, whole (Carnation)	½ cup	170	53	10
Goat milk	1 cup	168	54	10
Human milk	1 cup	168	43	8
Lowfat, 1%	1 cup	102	28	3
Lowfat, 2%	1 cup	121	35	5
Skim	1 cup	86	4	Tr
Skim, dry	¼ cup	109	1	Tr
Soybean milk	1 cup	79	57	5
Soybean Milk (Soy Moo)	1 cup	140	39	6
Whole, 3.3% fat	1 cup	150	48	8
Whole, 3.5% fat	1 cup	150	48	8
Whole, 3.7% fat	1 cup	157	52	9

MILK BEVERAGES

Note: Unless otherwise noted, all milk drinks are listed as prepared with 1 cup of whole milk.

Chocolate (Ovaltine)	1 cup	227	36	9
Chocolate syrup	1 cup	232	31	8
Egg nog, nonalcoholic	1 cup	342	50	19
Hot Cocoa, prep. w/water (Carnation)	1 cup	110	8	1
Hot Cocoa, 70 Calorie, prep. w/water (Carnation)	1 cup	70	1	Tr

Product	Portion	Calories	Percent Calories from Fat	Fat Grams

MILK AND MILK BEVERAGES

MILK BEVERAGES

Note: Unless otherwise noted, all milk drinks are listed as prepared with 1 cup of whole milk.

Product	Portion	Calories	Percent Calories from Fat	Fat Grams
Hot Cocoa, Sugar Free, prep. w/water (Swiss Miss)	1 cup	50	18	1
Instant Breakfast, Vanilla (Carnation)	1 cup	130	0	0
Malted milk	1 cup	236	38	10
Malted Milk, Chocolate (Kraft)	1 cup	240	34	9
Milkshake, chocolate	1 cup	230	35	9

NUTS AND PEANUT BUTTER

Product	Portion	Calories	Percent Calories from Fat	Fat Grams
Almonds	1 oz	174	83	16
Beechnuts	1 oz	164	77	14
Brazil nuts	8 medium	186	92	19
Cashews, roasted	1 oz	163	77	14
Chestnuts, roasted	1 oz	57	2	Tr
Coconut, shredded, sweetened	1 oz	142	63	10
Hazelnuts (filberts)	1 oz	187	87	18
Hickory nuts	1 oz	187	87	18
Macadamia nuts	1 oz	204	97	22
Mixed Nuts (Planters)	1 oz	180	80	16

Product	Portion	Calories	Percent Calories from Fat	Fat Grams

NUTS AND PEANUT BUTTER

Product	Portion	Calories	Percent Calories from Fat	Fat Grams
Peanuts	1 oz	163	77	14
Peanut Butter (Jif)	2 tbsp	190	76	16
Peanut Butter (Skippy Super Chunk)	2 tbsp	190	81	17
Pecans	1 oz	190	90	19
Pignolias (pine nuts)	1 oz	146	86	14
Pistachios	1 oz	172	78	15
Walnuts, black	1 oz	172	84	16
Walnuts, English	1 oz	182	89	18

PANCAKES AND WAFFLES

Product	Portion	Calories	Percent Calories from Fat	Fat Grams
French toast	2 slices	310	41	14
Pancakes, Blueberry (Hungry Jack)	3	320	42	15
Pancakes, Buttermilk (Aunt Jemima)	3	250	14	4
Pancakes, Buttermilk (Hungry Jack)	3	240	41	11
Pancakes, Original (Aunt Jemima)	3	260	14	4
Potato pancakes	3	234	69	18
Waffles, from mix	2	420	26	12
Waffles, Blueberry, Toaster (Eggo)	2	260	35	10
Waffles, Nutri-Grain, Toaster (Eggo)	2	260	35	10
Waffles, Whole Wheat, Toaster (Roman Meal)	2	280	45	14

Product	Portion	Calories	Percent Calories from Fat	Fat Grams

PASTA

Note: All items in this category are cooked.

Product	Portion	Calories	Percent Calories from Fat	Fat Grams
Egg noodles	1 cup	200	9	2
Macaroni, cooked firm	1 cup	190	5	1
Macaroni, cooked tender	1 cup	155	6	1
Spaghetti, cooked firm	1 cup	190	5	1
Spaghetti, cooked tender	1 cup	155	6	1

PASTRIES

Product	Portion	Calories	Percent Calories from Fat	Fat Grams
Bear claw	1	250	54	15
Cinnamon Roll (Pillsbury)	1	230	35	9
Cream Puffs, Bavarian, frozen (Rich's)	1	146	49	8
Cream puffs, with custard	1	393	53	18
Danish Apple (Hostess)	1	360	50	20
Danish, Butterhorn (Hostess)	1	330	49	18
Danish, Raspberry (Hostess)	1	270	23	7
Donuts, Chocolate Coated (Hostess)	1	130	55	8
Donuts, Cinnamon (Hostess)	1	110	49	6

Product	Portion	Calories	Percent Calories from Fat	Fat Grams

PASTRIES

Product	Portion	Calories	Percent Calories from Fat	Fat Grams
Donuts, Krunch (Hostess)	1	110	33	4
Donuts, Old Fashioned (Hostess)	1	172	52	10
Donuts, Old Fashioned Glazed (Hostess)	1	230	47	12
Donuts, Powdered Sugar (Hostess)	1	110	41	5
Eclair, Chocolate, frozen (Rich's)	1	205	44	10
Popovers, homemade	1	90	40	4
Pop Tarts, Blueberry	1	210	21	5
Pop Tarts, Frosted Dutch Apple	1	210	26	6
Raisin bun	1	179	10	2
Streudel, Apple Cinnamon (Pillsbury)	1	187	43	9
Sweet roll	1	154	41	7
Toastettes, Apple	1	200	22	5
Toastettes, Brown Sugar Cinnamon	1	200	22	5

PIES

DESSERT PIES

Product	Portion	Calories	Percent Calories from Fat	Fat Grams
Apple (Banquet)	⅙ pie	253	39	11
Apple (Mrs. Smith's)	⅛ pie	390	39	17
Apple, Natural Juice (Mrs. Smith's)	⅐ pie	420	47	22

Product	Portion	Calories	Percent Calories from Fat	Fat Grams
PIES				
DESSERT PIES				
Apple, homemade	⅛ pie	282	38	12
Banana Cream (Banquet)	⅙ pie	177	51	10
Blueberry (Banquet)	⅙ pie	266	37	11
Blueberry (Mrs. Smith's)	⅛ pie	380	40	17
Blueberry, homemade	1 slice	387	39	17
Cherry (Banquet)	⅙ pie	252	39	11
Cherry (Mrs. Smith's)	⅛ pie	400	36	16
Cherry, Natural Juice (Mrs. Smith's)	⅐ pie	410	40	18
Cherry, homemade	1 slice	418	39	18
Chocolate Mint (Royal)	⅛ pie	260	52	15
Coconut Cream (Jell-O)	⅛ pie	260	59	17
Coconut Custard (Mrs. Smith's)	⅛ pie	330	41	15
Custard, homemade	⅛ pie	324	50	18
Lemon chiffon, homemade	⅛ pie	254	35	10
Lemon Cream (Banquet)	⅙ pie	173	47	9
Lemon meringue pie, homemade	⅙ pie	350	33	13
Mince, homemade	⅛ pie	320	39	14

Product	Portion	Calories	Percent Calories from Fat	Fat Grams

PIES

DESSERT PIES
  Peach
    (Mrs. Smith's) | ⅛ pie | 365 | 39 | 16
  Peach, homemade | ⅛ pie | 320 | 39 | 14
  Pecan
    (Mrs. Smith's) | ⅛ pie | 510 | 41 | 23
  Pumpkin (Banquet) | ⅙ pie | 197 | 37 | 8
  Pumpkin,
    homemade | 1 slice | 325 | 36 | 13
  Pumpkin Custard
    (Mrs. Smith's) | ⅛ pie | 310 | 32 | 11
  Rhubarb,
    homemade | ⅐ pie | 299 | 39 | 13
  Strawberry,
    homemade | ⅐ pie | 184 | 34 | 7
  Sweet potato,
    homemade | ⅛ pie | 243 | 48 | 13
SNACK PIES
  Apple (Hostess) | 1 pie | 403 | 45 | 20
  Blueberry
    (Hostess) | 1 pie | 391 | 46 | 20
  Cherry (Hostess) | 1 pie | 416 | 43 | 20
  Lemon (Hostess) | 1 pie | 416 | 45 | 21

PORK

Note: Fresh meat figures are for separable lean only, unless otherwise mentioned.

BACON	2 slices	73	74	6
Armour	2 slices	76	71	6
Oscar Mayer	2 slices	70	77	6

Product	Portion	Calories	Percent Calories from Fat	Fat Grams

PORK

Note: Fresh meat figures are for separable lean only, unless otherwise mentioned.

Product	Portion	Calories	Percent Calories from Fat	Fat Grams
Bacon Bits (Oscar Mayer)	½ oz	42	43	2
Brains, cooked	3½ oz	138	65	10
Breakfast Strips (Oscar Mayer)	2 strips	104	87	10
Brown 'n Serve Links (Jones)	2 links	110	82	10
Brown 'n Serve Patties (Jones)	2 patties	272	73	22
Canadian Bacon (Oscar Mayer)	2 oz	70	26	2
Chitterlings, raw	3½ oz	249	83	23
Chitterlings, cooked	3½ oz	303	86	29
Ears, cooked	1 ear	183	59	12
Feet, cooked	3½ oz	194	56	12
HAM				
Boneless (Armour Star)	3½ oz	144	44	7
Fresh, raw	3½ oz	131	34	5
Fresh, roasted	3½ oz	145	37	6
Canned (Krakus)	3½ oz	193	56	12
Canned (Oscar Mayer)	3½ oz	109	29	4
Ham Salad Spread (Oscar Mayer)	3½ oz	207	61	14
Ham patties	2 patties	406	80	36
Heart, braised	1 heart	191	33	7
Kidneys, braised	3½ oz	151	30	5
Liver, braised	3½ oz	219	45	11

Product	Portion	Calories	Percent Calories from Fat	Fat Grams

PORK

Note: Fresh meat figures are for separable lean only, unless otherwise mentioned.

Product	Portion	Calories	Percent Calories from Fat	Fat Grams
Loin, broiled	3½ oz	231	43	11
Loin, fried	3½ oz	266	54	16
Loin, roasted	3½ oz	240	49	13
Shank, roasted	3½ oz	215	46	11
Shoulder, roasted	3½ oz	244	55	15
Sirloin, broiled	3½ oz	244	52	14
Sirloin, roasted	3½ oz	236	50	13
Spareribs, braised, lean and fat	3½ oz	398	68	30
Spareribs, raw, lean and fat	3½ oz	284	73	23
Tenderloin, raw	3½ oz	112	16	2
Tenderloin, roasted	3½ oz	166	27	5
Tongue, braised	3½ oz	271	63	19
Top loin, braised	3½ oz	277	45	14
Top loin, broiled	3½ oz	258	52	15
Top loin, fried	3½ oz	257	54	15
Top loin, roasted	3½ oz	245	51	14

POTATO CHIPS AND SNACKS

Product	Portion	Calories	Percent Calories from Fat	Fat Grams
Cheez Curls (Planters)	1 oz	160	62	11
Corn Chips (Wise)	1 oz	160	56	10
Doo Dads (Nabisco)	1 oz	140	39	6
Popcorn, air popped	1 cup	30	3	Tr
Popcorn, popped in oil	1 cup	55	49	3

Product	Portion	Calories	Percent Calories from Fat	Fat Grams
POTATO CHIPS AND SNACKS				
Potato Chips (Wise)	1 oz	160	62	11
Potato Crunchies (Planters)	1 oz	142	51	8
Pretzels (Mr. Salty)	1 oz	110	8	1
Pretzels (Quinlan)	1 oz	105	1	Tr
Tortilla Chips (La Famous)	1 oz	140	45	7
PUDDING				
Banana Cream (Royal)	½ cup	160	23	4
Banana Cream, Instant (Jell-O)	½ cup	160	23	4
Banana Cream, Instant (Royal)	½ cup	180	25	5
Banana Cream, Sugar Free (Jell-O)	½ cup	88	20	2
Bread with raisins, homemade	½ cup	180	25	5
Butterscotch (Jell-O)	½ cup	170	21	4
Butterscotch (Royal)	½ cup	160	23	4
Butterscotch, Instant (Jell-O)	½ cup	160	23	4
Butterscotch, Instant (Royal)	½ cup	180	25	5
Chocolate (Jell-O)	½ cup	160	23	4
Chocolate (Rich's)	½ cup	188	43	9
Chocolate (Royal)	½ cup	180	20	4
Chocolate, homemade	½ cup	193	28	6

Product	Portion	Calories	Percent Calories from Fat	Fat Grams
PUDDING				
Chocolate, Instant (Jell-O)	½ cup	180	20	4
Chocolate, Instant (Royal)	½ cup	190	19	4
Chocolate, Reduced Calorie (D-Zerta)	½ cup	60	0	0
Chocolate Fudge, Instant (Jell-O)	½ cup	174	24	5
Chocolate, Sugar Free (Jell-O)	½ cup	100	27	3
Coconut Cream, Instant (Jell-O)	½ cup	178	32	6
Corn, homemade	½ cup	97	9	1
Custard (Jell-O Americana)	½ cup	160	28	5
Custard (Royal)	½ cup	150	30	5
Custard, homemade	½ cup	153	41	7
Flan (Royal)	½ cup	150	30	5
Key Lime Pie Filling (Royal)	½ cup	160	17	3
Lemon, Instant (Jell-O)	½ cup	170	21	4
Lemon, Instant (Royal)	½ cup	180	25	5
Milk Chocolate, Instant (Jell-O)	½ cup	178	25	5
Pineapple Cream, Instant (Jell-O)	½ cup	165	22	4
Pistachio, Instant (Jell-O)	½ cup	170	26	5
Pumpkin, homemade	½ cup	170	26	5

Product	Portion	Calories	Percent Calories from Fat	Fat Grams
PUDDING				
Rice (Jell-O)	½ cup	170	21	4
Rice with raisins, homemade	½ cup	246	22	6
Tapioca (Jell-O)	½ cup	160	23	4
Tapioca, from mix	½ cup	145	25	4
Vanilla (Jell-O)	½ cup	160	23	4
Vanilla (Royal)	½ cup	160	23	4
Vanilla, Reduced Calorie (D-Zerta)	½ cup	69	1	Tr
SALAD DRESSING				
REDUCED CALORIE				
Blue Cheese (Roka)	1 tbsp	14	64	1
Blue Cheese, Chunky (Kraft)	1 tbsp	30	60	2
Buttermilk (Wish-Bone)	1 tbsp	38	95	4
Cucumber, Creamy (Kraft)	1 tbsp	30	90	3
French	1 tbsp	22	20	<1
French (Kraft)	1 tbsp	25	72	2
French Style (Pritikin)	1 tbsp	10	0	0
Italian	1 tbsp	16	84	<2
Italian (Kraft)	1 tbsp	6	0	0
Italian (Walden Farms)	1 tbsp	9	10	Tr
Italian, Creamy (Kraft)	1 tbsp	25	72	2

Product	Portion	Calories	Percent Calories from Fat	Fat Grams

SALAD DRESSING

REDUCED CALORIE

Product	Portion	Calories	Percent Calories from Fat	Fat Grams
Italian, Oil-Free (Kraft)	1 tbsp	4	0	0
Italian, Sugar-Free (Walden Farms)	1 tbsp	6	15	Tr
Ranch (Walden Farms)	1 tbsp	35	51	2
Russian	1 tbsp	23	20	< 1
Russian (Kraft)	1 tbsp	30	30	1
Thousand Island	1 tbsp	24	56	< 2
Thousand Island (Kraft)	1 tbsp	30	60	2
Vinaigrette (Herb Magic)	1 tbsp	6	0	0
Zesty Tomato (Herb Magic)	1 tbsp	14	0	0

REGULAR

Product	Portion	Calories	Percent Calories from Fat	Fat Grams
Bacon & Buttermilk (Kraft)	1 tbsp	80	90	8
Blue Cheese (Roka)	1 tbsp	60	90	6
Blue Cheese, Chunky (Kraft)	1 tbsp	70	77	6
Blue cheese, homemade	1 tbsp	77	94	8
Blue Cheese & Herbs, from mix (Good Seasons)	1 tbsp	72	100	8
Buttermilk, Creamy (Kraft)	1 tbsp	80	90	8

Product	Portion	Calories	Percent Calories from Fat	Fat Grams

SALAD DRESSING

REGULAR
Buttermilk, from mix (Good Seasons)	1 tbsp	58	93	6
Buttermilk & Chives, Creamy (Kraft)	1 tbsp	80	90	8
Caesar (Wish-Bone)	1 tbsp	78	92	8
Coleslaw (Kraft)	1 tbsp	70	77	6
Cucumber, Creamy (Kraft)	1 tbsp	70	100	8
Dijon, Creamy (Wish-Bone)	1 tbsp	62	87	6
Dijon Vinaigrette (Wish-Bone)	1 tbsp	61	89	6
French (Catalina)	1 tbsp	70	77	6
French (Kraft)	1 tbsp	60	90	6
French, Deluxe (Wish-Bone)	1 tbsp	59	92	6
French, homemade	1 tbsp	88	100	10
Garlic, Creamy (Kraft)	1 tbsp	50	90	5
Garlic, Creamy (Wish-Bone)	1 tbsp	74	97	8
Garlic & Herbs, from mix (Good Seasons)	1 tbsp	84	96	9
Italian	1 tbsp	69	91	7
Italian, Creamy (Kraft)	1 tbsp	60	90	6

Product	Portion	Calories	Percent Calories from Fat	Fat Grams

SALAD DRESSING

REGULAR

Product	Portion	Calories	Percent Calories from Fat	Fat Grams
Italian, Creamy (Wish-Bone)	1 tbsp	56	80	5
Italian Herbal Classic (Wish-Bone)	1 tbsp	70	90	7
Oil & Vinegar (Kraft)	1 tbsp	70	90	7
Oil & vinegar, homemade	1 tbsp	72	100	8
Oil & Vinegar, Red Wine (Kraft)	1 tbsp	50	72	4
Onion & Chives, Creamy (Kraft)	1 tbsp	70	90	7
Ranch (Kraft)	1 tbsp	80	90	8
Romano & Parmesan (Wish-Bone)	1 tbsp	89	91	9
Russian (Kraft)	1 tbsp	60	75	5
Russian (Wish-Bone)	1 tbsp	47	57	3
Sesame seed	1 tbsp	68	93	7
Thousand Island (Kraft)	1 tbsp	60	75	5
Thousand Island (Wish-Bone)	1 tbsp	69	65	5
Thousand Island & Bacon (Kraft)	1 tbsp	60	90	6

Product	Portion	Calories	Percent Calories from Fat	Fat Grams
SANDWICH MEATS				
Bar-B-Q Loaf (Oscar Mayer)	2 oz	100	54	6
Barbecue Loaf (Armour)	2 oz	100	54	6
Beef (Buddig)	2 oz	80	45	4
Beef, Italian Style (Oscar Mayer)	2 oz	60	45	3
Beerwurst	2 oz	183	84	17
BOLOGNA				
Beef	2 oz	178	81	16
Beef (Armour)	2 oz	200	81	18
Beef (Health Valley)	2 oz	177	86	17
Beef (Oscar Mayer)	2 oz	180	80	16
Beef, Garlic Flavored (Oscar Mayer)	2 oz	178	81	16
Beef, Lower Salt (Armour)	2 oz	180	80	16
Beef & Pork	2 oz	178	81	16
Berliner	2 oz	130	69	10
Bologna & Cheese (Oscar Mayer)	2 oz	180	85	17
Chicken Bologna (Health Valley)	2 oz	170	90	17
Chicken Bologna (Tyson)	2 oz	130	69	10
Lebanon Bologna	2 oz	128	49	7
Pork Bologna	2 oz	140	77	12

Product	Portion	Calories	Percent Calories from Fat	Fat Grams
SANDWICH MEATS				
BOLOGNA				
Turkey Bologna	2 oz	110	65	8
Turkey Bologna (Armour)	2 oz	110	65	8
Braunschweiger (Oscar Mayer)	2 oz	192	84	18
Chicken (Buddig)	2 oz	100	54	6
Chicken Roll, Breast (Tyson)	2 oz	89	51	5
Chicken roll, light meat	2 oz	60	45	3
Chicken spread	2 oz	110	49	6
Corned Beef (Buddig)	2 oz	80	45	4
Corned Beef (Oscar Mayer)	2 oz	53	4	Tr
Corned beef, canned	2 oz	142	51	8
Corned beef loaf	2 oz	92	39	4
Dried beef	2 oz	94	19	2
Dutch Brand Loaf	2 oz	136	66	10
Ham (Buddig)	2 oz	100	54	6
Ham, Chopped (Oscar Mayer)	2 oz	110	65	8
Ham, Cracked Black Pepper (Oscar Mayer)	2 oz	64	4	Tr
Ham & Cheese Loaf (Oscar Mayer)	2 oz	150	72	12
Ham and cheese spread	2 oz	138	65	10

Product	Portion	Calories	Percent Calories from Fat	Fat Grams
SANDWICH MEATS				
Pickle & Pimiento Loaf (Oscar Mayer)	2 oz	139	55	8
Picnic loaf	2 oz	132	61	9
Pork, sliced	2 oz	320	96	34
Poultry salad spread	2 oz	114	63	8
SALAMI				
Beef	2 oz	148	79	13
Cotto (Oscar Mayer)	2 oz	135	67	10
Cotto, Beef (Oscar Mayer)	2 oz	112	60	8
Genoa (Armour)	2 oz	220	82	20
Hard (Armour)	2 oz	240	75	20
Hard (Oscar Mayer)	2 oz	204	79	18
Salami for Beer (Oscar Mayer)	2 oz	135	80	12
Turkey Cotto Salami (Armour)	2 oz	90	55	6
Turkey Cotto Salami (Louis Rich)	2 oz	104	69	8
Turkey Cotto Salami (Oscar Mayer)	2 oz	104	69	8
Sandwich Spread (Oscar Mayer)	2 oz	134	67	10
Spiced Luncheon Meat (Armour)	2 oz	187	77	16

Product	Portion	Calories	Percent Calories from Fat	Fat Grams
SANDWICH MEATS				
Turkey (Buddig)	2 oz	100	54	6
Turkey Breast, Barbecued (Louis Rich)	2 oz	76	24	2
Turkey Breast, Roasted (Louis Rich)	2 oz	72	25	2
Turkey Breast, Smoked (Louis Rich)	2 oz	70	26	2
Turkey Ham (Armour)	2 oz	70	26	2
Turkey Ham (Buddig)	2 oz	80	45	4
Turkey Ham (Louis Rich)	2 oz	68	26	2
Turkey Loaf, breast meat	2 oz	62	15	1
Turkey Pastrami (Armour)	2 oz	70	32	<3
Turkey Pastrami (Louis Rich)	2 oz	66	33	2
Turkey roll, light meat	2 oz	83	44	4
Turkey roll, light & dark meat	2 oz	84	43	4
Turkey Roll, White (Magic Slice)	2 oz	80	34	3
Turkey Roll, White & Dark (Magic Slice)	2 oz	80	34	3

Product	Portion	Calories	Percent Calories from Fat	Fat Grams
SAUSAGE				
Beef, smoked	1 link	134	81	12
Beef Smokies (Oscar Mayer)	1 link	122	81	11
Blood sausage	2 oz	214	84	20
Bratwurst	1 link	256	77	22
Breakfast Patties, Pork (Jones)	2 oz	136	73	11
Breakfast Sausage, Turkey (Bil Mar Foods)	2 oz	116	62	8
Brotwurst	1 link	226	80	20
Brown & Serve Links (Jones)	2 links	110	82	10
Brown & Serve Patties (Jones)	2 oz	136	73	11
Cheese Smokies (Oscar Mayer)	1 link	127	78	11
Chorizo	1 link	265	78	23
Country style	2 oz	200	72	16
Honey roll sausage	2 oz	104	52	6
Italian sausage	1 link	217	71	17
Kielbasa	2 oz	180	80	16
Knockwurst	1 link	209	82	19
Little Friers (Oscar Mayer)	2 links	153	83	14
Mortadella	2 oz	176	72	14
New England Brand, pork & beef	2 oz	9	40	4
Pepperoni (Armour)	2 oz	260	76	22
Pork & beef, smoked	1 link	229	83	21

Product	Portion	Calories	Percent Calories from Fat	Fat Grams
SAUSAGE				
Pork Sausage (Armour)	2 oz	220	90	22
Sausage Patties (Oscar Mayer)	1 patty	125	79	11
Smokie Links (Oscar Mayer)	1 link	124	80	11
Summer sausage	2 oz	196	73	16
Summer Sausage (Oscar Mayer)	2 oz	175	87	17
Summer Sausage, Beef (Oscar Mayer)	2 oz	175	77	15
Turkey Breakfast Sausage (Louis Rich)	2 oz	118	61	8
Turkey Smoked Sausage (Louis Rich)	2 oz	110	65	8
Turkey Summer Sausage (Louis Rich)	2 oz	104	69	8
Vienna Sausage (Armour)	2 oz	180	85	17
SOUP				

Note: Unless otherwise specified, canned soups are condensed and prepared with water.

CANNED SOUP				
Bean with bacon	8 fl oz	173	31	6

Product	Portion	Calories	Percent Calories from Fat	Fat Grams

SOUP

Note: Unless otherwise specified, canned soups are condensed and prepared with water.

CANNED SOUP

Product	Portion	Calories	Percent Calories from Fat	Fat Grams
Bean with Bacon, Special Request (Campbell's)	8 fl oz	120	30	4
Bean with frankfurters	8 fl oz	187	39	7
Bean with ham, chunky	8 fl oz	231	35	9
Beef (Campbell's)	8 fl oz	71	19	<2
Beef, chunky, rts*	8 fl oz	171	26	5
Beef Broth (College Inn)	8 fl oz	18	0	0
Beef Broth, rts (Health Valley)	8 fl oz	20	0	0
Beef and mushroom	8 fl oz	72	38	3
Beef noodle	8 fl oz	84	32	3
Beef Noodle (Campbell's)	8 fl oz	70	39	3
Beef Noodle, Homestyle (Campbell's)	8 fl oz	80	34	3
Black bean	8 fl oz	116	12	<2
Black Bean (Campbell's)	8 fl oz	110	16	2
Borscht (Gold's)	8 fl oz	100	0	0

* rts = Ready-to-serve.

Product	Portion	Calories	Percent Calories from Fat	Fat Grams

SOUP

Note: Unless otherwise specified, canned soups are condensed and prepared with water.

CANNED SOUP

Product	Portion	Calories	Percent Calories from Fat	Fat Grams
Cauliflower	8 fl oz	68	26	2
Cheddar Cheese (Campbell's)	8 fl oz	130	55	8
Cheese	8 fl oz	155	64	11
Cheese, prepared with milk	8 fl oz	230	59	15
Chicken, chunky, rts*	8 fl oz	178	35	7
Chicken Alphabet (Campbell's)	8 fl oz	70	26	2
Chicken and dumplings	8 fl oz	97	56	6
Chicken broth	8 fl oz	39	23	1
Chicken Broth, rts (College Inn)	8 fl oz	35	77	3
Chicken Broth, rts (Pritikin)	7 fl oz	14	0	0
Chicken Broth and Noodles (Campbell's)	8 fl oz	60	30	2
Chicken Broth with Rice (Campbell's)	8 fl oz	44	20	1
Chicken gumbo	8 fl oz	56	23	1
Chicken Gumbo (Campbell's)	8 fl oz	60	30	2

* rts = Ready-to-serve.

Product	Portion	Calories	Percent Calories from Fat	Fat Grams

SOUP

Note: Unless otherwise specified, canned soups are condensed and prepared with water.

CANNED SOUP

Product	Portion	Calories	Percent Calories from Fat	Fat Grams
Chicken Gumbo (Campbell's)	8 fl oz	60	30	2
Chicken Gumbo rts* (Pritikin)	7⅜ fl oz	60	15	1
Chicken 'N Dumplings (Campbell's)	8 fl oz	80	34	3
Chicken noodle	8 fl oz	75	30	<3
Chicken Noodle (Campbell's)	8 fl oz	70	26	2
Chicken noodle, chunky, rts	8 fl oz	180	30	6
Chicken noodle with meatballs	8 fl oz	99	36	4
Chicken NoodleOs (Campbell's)	8 fl oz	70	26	2
Chicken with Ribbon Pasta, rts (Pritikin)	7¼ fl oz	60	0	Tr
Chicken rice	8 fl oz	60	30	2
Chicken Rice (Campbell's)	8 fl oz	60	30	2
Chicken rice, chunky, rts	8 fl oz	127	21	3

* rts = Ready-to-serve.

Product	Portion	Calories	Percent Calories from Fat	Fat Grams

SOUP

Note: Unless otherwise specified, canned soups are condensed and prepared with water.

CANNED SOUP

Product	Portion	Calories	Percent Calories from Fat	Fat Grams
Chicken and Stars (Campbell's)	8 fl oz	55	33	2
Chicken vegetable	8 fl oz	74	36	3
Chicken Vegetable (Campbell's)	8 fl oz	70	39	3
Chicken Vegetable, rts* (Pritikin)	7¼ fl oz	60	2	Tr
Chicken vegetable, chunky	8 fl oz	167	27	5
Chili beef	8 fl oz	169	35	7
Chili Beef (Campbell's)	8 fl oz	130	35	5
Clam chowder, Manhattan	8 fl oz	78	23	2
Clam Chowder, Manhattan (Campbell's)	8 fl oz	70	26	2
Clam chowder, Manhattan, chunky, rts	8 fl oz	133	20	3
Clam chowder, New England	8 fl oz	95	28	3

* rts = Ready-to-serve.

Product	Portion	Calories	Percent Calories from Fat	Fat Grams

SOUP

Note: Unless otherwise specified, canned soups are condensed and prepared with water.

CANNED SOUP

Product	Portion	Calories	Percent Calories from Fat	Fat Grams
Clam Chowder, New England (Campbell's)	8 fl oz	80	34	3
Clam chowder, New England, prepared with milk	8 fl oz	163	39	7
Consomme, beef	8 fl oz	29	0	0
Crab, rts*	8 fl oz	76	24	2
Cream of asparagus	8 fl oz	87	41	4
Cream of Asparagus (Campbell's)	8 fl oz	90	40	4
Cream of asparagus, prepared with milk	8 fl oz	161	45	8
Cream of Celery (Campbell's)	8 fl oz	100	63	7
Cream of celery, prepared with milk	8 fl oz	165	55	10

* rts = Ready-to-serve.

Product	Portion	Calories	Percent Calories from Fat	Fat Grams

SOUP

Note: Unless otherwise specified, canned soups are condensed and prepared with water.

CANNED SOUP

Product	Portion	Calories	Percent Calories from Fat	Fat Grams
Cream of chicken	8 fl oz	116	54	7
Cream of Chicken (Campbell's)	8 fl oz	110	57	7
Cream of chicken, prepared with milk	8 fl oz	191	52	11
Cream of mushroom	8 fl oz	129	63	9
Cream of Mushroom (Campbell's)	8 fl oz	129	63	9
Cream of mushroom, prepared with milk	8 fl oz	203	62	14
Cream of Onion (Campbell's)	8 fl oz	100	45	5
Cream of potato	8 fl oz	73	30	2
Cream of Potato (Campbell's)	8 fl oz	70	39	3
Cream of potato, prepared with milk	8 fl oz	148	36	6
Cream of shrimp	8 fl oz	90	50	5
Cream of Shrimp (Campbell's)	8 fl oz	90	60	6

Product	Portion	Calories	Percent Calories from Fat	Fat Grams

SOUP

Note: Unless otherwise specified, canned soups are condensed and prepared with water.

CANNED SOUP

Product	Portion	Calories	Percent Calories from Fat	Fat Grams
Cream of shrimp, prepared with milk	8 fl oz	165	49	9
Cream of Shrimp, prepared with milk (Campbell's)	8 fl oz	160	56	10
Cream of Tomato, prepared with milk (Campbell's)	8 fl oz	160	34	6
Curly Noodle with Chicken (Campbell's)	8 fl oz	67	31	2
Escarole, rts*	8 fl oz	27	67	2
French Onion (Campbell's)	8 fl oz	60	30	2
Gazpacho, rts	8 fl oz	57	32	2
Green Pea (Campbell's)	8 fl oz	160	17	3
Lentil with ham	8 fl oz	140	19	3
Meatball Alphabet (Campbell's)	8 fl oz	100	36	4

* rts = Ready-to-serve.

Product	Portion	Calories	Percent Calories from Fat	Fat Grams

SOUP

Note: Unless otherwise specified, canned soups are condensed and prepared with water.

CANNED SOUP

Product	Portion	Calories	Percent Calories from Fat	Fat Grams
Minestrone	8 fl oz	83	33	3
Minestrone (Campbell's)	8 fl oz	80	23	2
Minestrone, chunky	8 fl oz	127	21	3
Mushroom (Pritikin)	7⅜ fl oz	60	2	Tr
Mushroom, Golden (Campbell's)	8 fl oz	80	34	3
Mushroom with beef stock	8 fl oz	85	42	4
Nacho Cheese (Campbell's)	8 fl oz	100	72	8
Navy Bean rts* (Pritikin)	7⅜ fl oz	130	1	Tr
Noodles and Ground Beef (Campbell's)	8 fl oz	90	40	4
Onion	8 fl oz	57	27	2
Oyster stew	8 fl oz	59	61	4
Oyster Stew (Campbell's)	8 fl oz	80	56	5

* rts = Ready-to-serve.

Product	Portion	Calories	Percent Calories from Fat	Fat Grams

SOUP

Note: Unless otherwise specified, canned soups are condensed and prepared with water.

CANNED SOUP

Product	Portion	Calories	Percent Calories from Fat	Fat Grams
Oyster stew, prepared with milk	8 fl oz	134	54	8
Oyster Stew, prepared with milk (Campbell's)	8 fl oz	150	54	9
Pea, green	8 fl oz	164	16	3
Pea, green, prepared with milk	8 fl oz	239	26	7
Pepperpot	8 fl oz	103	44	5
Pepperpot (Campbell's)	8 fl oz	90	40	4
Schav, rts* (Gold's)	8 fl oz	25	0	0
Scotch broth	8 fl oz	80	29	<3
Scotch Broth (Campbell's)	8 fl oz	80	34	3
Stockpot	8 fl oz	100	36	4
Tomato	8 fl oz	86	21	2
Tomato (Campbell's)	8 fl oz	90	20	2
Tomato, rts (Pritikin)	7¼ fl oz	70	0	0

* rts = Ready-to-serve.

Product	Portion	Calories	Percent Calories from Fat	Fat Grams

SOUP

Note: Unless otherwise specified, canned soups are condensed and prepared with water.

CANNED SOUP

Product	Portion	Calories	Percent Calories from Fat	Fat Grams
Tomato, prepared with milk	8 fl oz	160	34	6
Tomato, prepared with milk (Campbell's)	8 fl oz	160	34	6
Tomato beef with noodle	8 fl oz	140	26	4
Tomato bisque	8 fl oz	123	18	<3
Tomato Bisque (Campbell's)	8 fl oz	120	23	3
Tomato bisque, prepared with milk	8 fl oz	198	32	7
Tomato rice	8 fl oz	120	23	3
Tomato Rice, Old Fashioned (Campbell's)	8 fl oz	110	16	2
Turkey, chunky, rts*	8 fl oz	136	26	4
Turkey noodle	8 fl oz	69	26	2
Turkey Noodle (Campbell's)	8 fl oz	70	39	3
Turkey vegetable	8 fl oz	74	36	3
Turkey Vegetable (Campbell's)	8 fl oz	70	39	3

* rts = Ready-to-serve.

Product	Portion	Calories	Percent Calories from Fat	Fat Grams

SOUP

Note: Unless otherwise specified, canned soups are condensed and prepared with water.

CANNED SOUP

Product	Portion	Calories	Percent Calories from Fat	Fat Grams
Vegetable (Campbell's)	8 fl oz	90	20	2
Vegetable rts* (Pritikin)	7¼ fl oz	70	0	0
Vegetable, chunky, rts	8 fl oz	122	30	4
Vegetable, Old-Fashioned (Campbell's)	8 fl oz	60	30	2
Vegetable, vegetarian	8 fl oz	72	25	2
Vegetable, Vegetarian (Campbell's)	8 fl oz	90	20	2
Vegetable beef	8 fl oz	79	23	2
Vegetable Beef (Campbell's)	8 fl oz	70	26	2
Vegetable with beef broth	8 fl oz	81	22	2
Vichyssoise	8 fl oz	148	36	6
Won Ton (Campbell's)	8 fl oz	40	23	1
DRY SOUPS				
Bean with bacon	8 fl oz	105	17	2
Beef bouillon	8 fl oz	19	47	1
Beef bouillon, cubed	8 fl oz	6	15	Tr

* rts = Ready-to-serve.

Product	Portion	Calories	Percent Calories from Fat	Fat Grams

SOUP

DRY SOUPS

Product	Portion	Calories	Percent Calories from Fat	Fat Grams
Beef noodle	8 fl oz	41	22	1
Cauliflower	8 fl oz	68	26	2
Chicken bouillon, cubed	8 fl oz	9	10	Tr
Chicken broth	8 fl oz	21	43	1
Chicken noodle	8 fl oz	53	17	1
Chicken rice	8 fl oz	60	15	1
Chicken vegetable	8 fl oz	49	18	1
Clam chowder, Manhattan	8 fl oz	65	28	2
Clam chowder, New England	8 fl oz	95	38	4
Consomme	8 fl oz	17	5	Tr
Cream of asparagus	8 fl oz	59	31	2
Cream of celery	8 fl oz	63	29	2
Cream of chicken	8 fl oz	107	42	5
Cream of vegetable	8 fl oz	105	51	6
Leek	8 fl oz	71	25	2
Minestrone	8 fl oz	79	23	2
Mushroom	8 fl oz	96	47	5
Onion	8 fl oz	28	32	1
Oxtail	8 fl oz	71	38	3
Split pea	8 fl oz	133	14	2
Tomato	8 fl oz	102	18	2
Tomato vegetable	8 fl oz	55	16	1
Vegetable beef	8 fl oz	53	17	1

Product	Portion	Calories	Percent Calories from Fat	Fat Grams
TOMATOES AND TOMATO PRODUCTS				
Canned, Whole (Contadina)	½ cup	25	4	Tr
Fresh, boiled	½ cup	30	3	Tr
Marinara Sauce (Ragu)	½ cup	90	40	4
Paste (Contadina)	¼ cup	50	2	Tr
Puree (Contadina)	¼ cup	20	0	0
Raw	1 medium	24	4	Tr
Spaghetti Sauce (Prego)	½ cup	140	39	6
Spaghetti Sauce with Mushrooms (Prego)	½ cup	140	32	5
Spaghetti Sauce with Mushrooms (Prego)	⅓ cup	140	32	5
Spaghetti Sauce (Pritikin)	½ cup	60	0	0
Spaghetti Sauce with Mushrooms (Pritikin)	½ cup	60	0	0
Spaghetti Sauce, Gardenstyle with Mushrooms & Onions (Ragu)	½ cup	80	20	2
Spaghetti Sauce, Gardenstyle with Extra Tomatoes, Garlic & Onions (Ragu)	½ cup	80	20	2

Product	Portion	Calories	Percent Calories from Fat	Fat Grams

TOMATOES AND TOMATO PRODUCTS

Product	Portion	Calories	Percent Calories from Fat	Fat Grams
Spaghetti Sauce, Homestyle Flavored with Meat (Ragu)	½ cup	70	26	2
Spaghetti Sauce, Homestyle Plain (Ragu)	½ cup	70	26	2
Spaghetti Sauce, Homestyle with Mushrooms (Ragu)	½ cup	70	26	2
Spaghetti Sauce, Thick & Hearty, Plain (Ragu)	½ cup	110	33	4
Spaghetti Sauce, Thick & Zesty with Meat (Ragu)	½ cup	100	36	4
Spaghetti Sauce, Thick & Zesty with Mushrooms (Ragu)	½ cup	110	41	5

TURKEY

ROASTERS

Product	Portion	Calories	Percent Calories from Fat	Fat Grams
All meat & skin	3½ oz	208	43	10
All meat only	3½ oz	170	26	5
Dark meat & skin	3½ oz	221	47	12
Dark meat only	3½ oz	187	34	7
Light meat & skin	3½ oz	197	37	8
Light meat only	3½ oz	157	17	3

Product	Portion	Calories	Percent Calories from Fat	Fat Grams
TURKEY				
PARTS				
Breast with skin, raw	3½ oz	157	38	7
Breast with skin, roasted	3½ oz	189	38	8
Giblets, simmered	3½ oz	167	27	5
Leg with skin, raw	3½ oz	138	42	6
Leg with skin, roasted	3½ oz	202	45	10
Liver, simmered	3½ oz	169	32	6
Neck, simmered	1 neck	274	36	11
Skin only, roasted	3½ oz	473	80	42
Wing with skin, raw	3½ oz	200	47	11
Wing with skin, roasted	3½ oz	221	45	11
TURKEY PRODUCTS				
Breast, Barbecued (Louis Rich)	3½ oz	137	30	5
Breast, Oven Roasted (Louis Rich)	3½ oz	105	21	<3
Breast, Hickory Smoked (Louis Rich)	3½ oz	123	3	4
Breast Tenderloins (Louis Rich)	3½ oz	145	9	<2
Canned	3½ oz	153	39	7
Diced, seasoned	3½ oz	137	46	7

Product	Portion	Calories	Percent Calories from Fat	Fat Grams
TURKEY				
TURKEY PRODUCTS				
Drumsticks, cooked				
(Louis Rich)	3½ oz	193	49	11
Ground Turkey				
(Louis Rich)	3½ oz	213	52	12
Patties				
(Louis Rich)	1 patty	266	58	17
Thighs, cooked				
(Louis Rich)	3½ oz	228	55	14
Wing Drumettes				
(Louis Rich)	3½ oz	182	38	8
Wings				
(Land O' Lakes)	3½ oz	140	39	6

VEAL

Note: Figures are for lean and fat unless otherwise noted.

Product	Portion	Calories	Percent Calories from Fat	Fat Grams
Arm steak, cooked	3½ oz	298	57	19
Blade, cooked	3½ oz	276	55	17
Cutlet, breaded & fried	3½ oz	319	42	15
Cutlet, broiled	3½ oz	216	44	11
Flank, stewed	3½ oz	390	74	32
Foreshank, stewed	3½ oz	216	42	10
Loin, broiled	3½ oz	234	51	13
Loin chop, cooked	3½ oz	421	77	36
Plate, stewed	3½ oz	303	62	21
Rib, roasted	3½ oz	269	54	16

Product	Portion	Calories	Percent Calories from Fat	Fat Grams

VEGETABLES

Note: All vegetables are cooked unless otherwise specified.

FRESH

Product	Portion	Calories	Percent Calories from Fat	Fat Grams
Alfalfa sprouts, raw	½ cup	5	18	Tr
Artichoke	1 medium	53	2	Tr
Asparagus	½ cup	22	4	Tr
Asparagus, canned	½ cup	24	19	< 1
Avocado, California	1 medium	306	88	30
Avocado, Florida	1 medium	339	72	27
Bamboo shoots, raw	½ cup	21	4	Tr
Beans				
Black-eyed peas	½ cup	100	1	Tr
Broad (fava)	½ cup	93	1	Tr
Chick-peas (garbanzo)	½ cup	134	13	2
Kidney	½ cup	112	1	Tr
Lima	½ cup	115	1	Tr
Mung	½ cup	107	1	Tr
Pinto	½ cup	117	1	Tr
Soybeans	½ cup	149	48	8
White	½ cup	125	1	Tr
Bean sprouts, raw	½ cup	16	6	Tr
Beets	½ cup	26	3	Tr
Beets, raw	½ cup	30	3	Tr
Beet greens	½ cup	20	5	Tr
Broccoli	½ cup	23	4	Tr
Broccoli florets	½ cup	23	4	Tr
Broccoli, raw	½ cup	12	1	Tr

Product	Portion	Calories	Percent Calories from Fat	Fat Grams

VEGETABLES

Note: All vegetables are cooked unless otherwise specified.

FRESH

Product	Portion	Calories	Percent Calories from Fat	Fat Grams
Brussels sprouts	½ cup	30	3	Tr
Brussels sprouts, raw	½ cup	24	4	Tr
Burdock	½ cup	55	2	Tr
Cabbage				
Chinese	½ cup	10	1	Tr
Green	½ cup	10	1	Tr
Green, raw	½ cup	8	11	Tr
Red, raw	½ cup	10	1	Tr
Savoy, raw	½ cup	10	1	Tr
Carrot	½ cup	35	3	Tr
Carrot, raw	½ cup	24	4	Tr
Cauliflower	½ cup	15	6	Tr
Cauliflower, raw	½ cup	12	8	Tr
Celeriac	½ cup	29	3	Tr
Celery	½ cup	11	8	Tr
Celery, raw	½ cup	9	10	Tr
Chard	½ cup	18	5	Tr
Chard, raw	½ cup	3	30	Tr
Chicory, raw	½ cup	21	4	Tr
Collard greens	½ cup	13	7	Tr
Corn	½ cup	89	10	1
Corn, raw	½ cup	66	14	1
Corn salad, raw	½ cup	6	15	Tr
Cucumber, raw	½ cup	7	13	Tr
Dandelion greens	½ cup	17	5	Tr
Dandelion greens, raw	½ cup	13	7	Tr

Product	Portion	Calories	Percent Calories from Fat	Fat Grams

VEGETABLES

Note: All vegetables are cooked unless otherwise specified.

FRESH

Product	Portion	Calories	Percent Calories from Fat	Fat Grams
Dasheen (taro)	½ cup	94	1	Tr
Eggplant	½ cup	14	6	Tr
Eggplant, raw	½ cup	11	0	0
Endive, raw	½ cup	4	23	Tr
French beans	½ cup	114	4	Tr
Garden cress, raw	½ cup	8	11	Tr
Gingerroot, raw	½ cup	17	5	Tr
Green beans	½ cup	22	4	Tr
Kale	½ cup	2	4	Tr
Kale, raw	½ cup	17	5	Tr
Kohlrabi	½ cup	24	4	Tr
Leeks	½ cup	16	6	Tr
Lentils	½ cup	115	1	Tr
Lettuce				
Bibb, raw	2 leaves	2	0	0
Looseleaf, raw	½ cup	5	18	Tr
Romaine, raw	½ cup	4	23	Tr
Lotus root, raw	5 slices	23	4	Tr
Mushrooms	½ cup	21	4	Tr
Mushrooms, raw	½ cup	9	10	Tr
Mustard greens	½ cup	11	8	Tr
Mustard greens, raw	½ cup	7	13	Tr
Okra	½ cup	25	4	Tr
Okra, raw	½ cup	13	7	Tr
Onion	½ cup	29	3	Tr
Onion, raw	½ cup	27	3	Tr
Parsley, raw	½ cup	10	9	Tr

Product	Portion	Calories	Percent Calories from Fat	Fat Grams

VEGETABLES

Note: All vegetables are cooked unless otherwise specified.

FRESH

Product	Portion	Calories	Percent Calories from Fat	Fat Grams
Parsnips	½ cup	63	1	Tr
Parsnips, raw	½ cup	50	2	Tr
Peas	½ cup	67	1	Tr
Peas, raw	½ cup	63	1	Tr
Pepper				
Green, raw	½ cup	18	5	Tr
Red	½ cup	12	8	Tr
Red, raw	½ cup	18	5	Tr
Potatoes				
Au gratin	½ cup	160	51	9
Baked, with skin	1 potato	220	0	Tr
Boiled, without skin	1 potato	116	1	Tr
French fries	10	109	33	4
Hash browns	½ cup	163	61	11
Mashed	½ cup	111	32	4
Scalloped	½ cup	105	43	5
Radishes, raw	½ cup	8	0	0
Rhubarb, raw	½ cup	15	6	Tr
Rutabaga, raw	½ cup	29	3	Tr
Shallots, raw	1 tbsp	7	0	0
Spinach	½ cup	21	4	Tr
Spinach, raw	½ cup	6	15	Tr
Split peas	½ cup	116	1	Tr
Squash				
Acorn, baked	½ cup	57	2	Tr
Butternut, mashed	½ cup	47	2	Tr

Product	Portion	Calories	Percent Calories from Fat	Fat Grams

VEGETABLES

Note: All vegetables are cooked unless otherwise specified.

FRESH
Squash

Product	Portion	Calories	Percent Calories from Fat	Fat Grams
Hubbard, mashed	½ cup	35	3	Tr
Spaghetti, baked	½ cup	35	3	Tr
Sweet potato	½ cup	118	1	Tr
Taro	½ cup	94	1	Tr
Tomato				
Green, raw	1	30	3	Tr
Red, boiled	½ cup	30	3	Tr
Red, raw	1	24	4	Tr
Red, stewed	½ cup	34	3	Tr
Turnip	½ cup	14	6	Tr
Turnip greens	½ cup	15	6	Tr
Watercress, raw	½ cup	2	45	Tr
Zucchini, raw	½ cup	9	10	Tr

CANNED

Product	Portion	Calories	Percent Calories from Fat	Fat Grams
Asparagus	½ cup	17	5	Tr
Bamboo shoots	½ cup	13	7	Tr
Beans				
Baked, plain	½ cup	118	8	1
Baked, with beef	½ cup	161	28	5
French style	½ cup	18	5	Tr
Kidney	½ cup	113	1	Tr
Lima	½ cup	109	1	Tr
Snap	½ cup	13	7	Tr
Beets, Harvard (Libby)	½ cup	80	0	0

Product	Portion	Calories	Percent Calories from Fat	Fat Grams

VEGETABLES

Note: All vegetables are cooked unless otherwise specified.

CANNED
Beets, Harvard (Seneca)	½ cup	80	0	0
Beets, Pickled (Libby)	½ cup	35	0	0
Carrots	½ cup	17	5	Tr
Chilies, jalapeño	½ cup	17	21	Tr
Corn	½ cup	66	11	<1
Hominy, white	½ cup	70	9	<1
Hominy, yellow	½ cup	65	8	<1
Mushrooms	½ cup	19	9	<1
Onion	½ cup	21	4	Tr
Peas	½ cup	59	5	Tr
Peas & Carrots (Libby)	½ cup	50	0	0
Pimientos	¼ cup	20	0	0
Pumpkin	½ cup	41	7	Tr
Sweet potatoes	½ cup	92	2	Tr
FROZEN				
Artichoke Hearts (Birds Eye)	½ cup	32	3	Tr
Beans				
Bavarian Style (Birds Eye)	½ cup	98	46	5
French Style	½ cup	26	3	Tr
Green Beans, Whole (Birds Eye)	½ cup	30	3	Tr
Italian Style	½ cup	31	3	Tr
Lima, Baby (Birds Eye)	½ cup	127	1	Tr

Product	Portion	Calories	Percent Calories from Fat	Fat Grams

VEGETABLES

Note: All vegetables are cooked unless otherwise specified.

CANNED
  Beans
   Snap | ½ cup | 18 | 5 | Tr
  Broccoli | ½ cup | 23 | 4 | Tr
  Broccoli with
   Cheese Sauce
   (Birds Eye) | ½ cup | 115 | 47 | 6
  Broccoli in
   Creamy Italian
   Cheese Sauce
   (Birds Eye) | ½ cup | 90 | 60 | 6
  Carrots | ½ cup | 26 | 3 | Tr
  Cauliflower
   (Birds Eye) | ½ cup | 20 | 5 | Tr
  Cauliflower in
   Cheese Sauce
   (Birds Eye) | ½ cup | 113 | 48 | 6
  Corn (Birds Eye) | ½ cup | 80 | 1 | Tr
  Corn Cob
   (Birds Eye) | 1 ear | 120 | 1 | Tr
  Corn Fritters
   (Mrs. Paul's) | 2 | 250 | 43 | 12
  Kale | ½ cup | 20 | 5 | Tr
  Mixed Vegetables
   Beans, French
    Style
    (Birds Eye) | ½ cup | 26 | 3 | Tr
   Beans, French
    Style with
    Almonds | ½ cup | 52 | 35 | 2

Product	Portion	Calories	Percent Calories from Fat	Fat Grams

VEGETABLES

Note: All vegetables are cooked unless otherwise specified.

CANNED
  Mixed Vegetables
    Beans, Italian
      Style
      (Birds Eye) | ½ cup | 31 | 3 | Tr

Product	Portion	Calories	Percent Calories from Fat	Fat Grams
Beans, Italian Style (Birds Eye)	½ cup	31	3	Tr
Beans, Onions, Red Peppers & Garlic	½ cup	18	5	Tr
Broccoli & Cauliflower (Birds Eye)	½ cup	20	0	0
Broccoli & Cauliflower in Cheese Sauce (Birds Eye)	½ cup	89	61	6
Broccoli, Cauliflower & Carrots (Birds Eye)	½ cup	22	4	Tr
Broccoli, Cauliflower & Carrots in Cheese Sauce (Birds Eye)	½ cup	99	45	5
Broccoli & Corn (Pillsbury)	½ cup	50	36	2
Broccoli, Corn & Red Peppers (Birds Eye)	½ cup	52	2	Tr

Product	Portion	Calories	Percent Calories from Fat	Fat Grams

VEGETABLES

Note: All vegetables are cooked unless otherwise specified.

CANNED
  Mixed Vegetables
    Broccoli, Green
      Beans, Onion
      & Red
      Peppers

Product	Portion	Calories	Percent Calories from Fat	Fat Grams
(Birds Eye)	½ cup	21	4	Tr

Broccoli, Red
      Pepper,
      Bamboo
      Shoots &
      Straw
      Mushrooms

(Birds Eye)	½ cup	19	5	Tr

Brussels Sprouts,
      Cauliflower &
      Carrots

(Birds Eye)	½ cup	27	3	Tr

Carrots &
      Cauliflower

(Pillsbury)	½ cup	60	45	3

Carrots, Peas &
      Onions

(Birds Eye)	½ cup	48	2	Tr

Chinese Style
      Vegetables

(Birds Eye)	½ cup	68	53	4

Chow Mein
      Style

(Birds Eye)	½ cup	89	40	4

Product	Portion	Calories	Percent Calories from Fat	Fat Grams

VEGETABLES

Note: All vegetables are cooked unless otherwise specified.

CANNED
  Mixed Vegetables

Product	Portion	Calories	Percent Calories from Fat	Fat Grams
Corn, Green Beans & Pasta Twists in Sauce (Birds Eye)	½ cup	107	42	5
Corn & Broccoli (Pillsbury)	½ cup	45	2	Tr
Green Beans, Bavarian Style & Spaetzle (Birds Eye)	½ cup	98	46	5
Italian Style Vegetables (Birds Eye)	½ cup	101	45	5
Japanese Style Vegetables (Birds Eye)	½ cup	88	41	4
Mandarin Style Vegetables (Birds Eye)	½ cup	86	42	4
Mixed Vegetables (Birds Eye)	½ cup	58	2	Tr
New England Style Vegetables (Birds Eye)	½ cup	124	44	6

Product	Portion	Calories	Percent Calories from Fat	Fat Grams

VEGETABLES

Note: All vegetables are cooked unless otherwise specified.

CANNED
  Mixed Vegetables
    Pasta
      Primavera
        (Birds Eye) | ½ cup | 122 | 37 | 5

	½ cup	122	37	5
Peas & Carrots	½ cup	48	2	Tr
Peas, Carrots & Onions (Birds Eye)	½ cup	48	2	Tr
Peas, Carrots & Onions in Butter Sauce (Le Sueur)	½ cup	80	34	3
Peas & Cauliflower (Pillsbury)	½ cup	30	3	Tr
Peas & Onions	½ cup	71	1	Tr
Peas & Onions in Cream Sauce (Birds Eye)	½ cup	137	33	5
Peas & Potatoes in Cream Sauce (Birds Eye)	½ cup	126	43	6
San Francisco Style Vegetables (Birds Eye)	½ cup	90	40	4

Product	Portion	Calories	Percent Calories from Fat	Fat Grams

VEGETABLES

Note: All vegetables are cooked unless otherwise specified.

CANNED
 Mixed Vegetables
  Spinach & Rice
   in Cheese
   Sauce

Product	Portion	Calories	Percent Calories from Fat	Fat Grams
(Birds Eye)	½ cup	170	37	7
Stir-Fry Style (Birds Eye)	½ cup	30	3	Tr
Stir-Fry, Chinese Style (Birds Eye)	½ cup	36	3	Tr
Mustard Greens	½ cup	14	6	Tr
Okra, cut	½ cup	25	0	0
Onion	½ cup	40	2	Tr
Onions in Cream Sauce (Birds Eye)	½ cup	100	54	6
Peas	½ cup	63	1	Tr
Peas in Cream Sauce (Birds Eye)	½ cup	118	46	6
Potatoes French fries	10	111	32	4
Hash browns	½ cup	170	48	9
Puffs	½ cup	138	46	7

YOGURT

Product	Portion	Calories	Percent Calories from Fat	Fat Grams
Apple (La Yogurt)	6 oz	190	19	4
Apple (Yoplait)	6 oz	190	14	3

Product	Portion	Calories	Percent Calories from Fat	Fat Grams
YOGURT				
Breakfast Yogurt, average of all fruit flavors (Yoplait)	6 oz	230	16	4
Banana (Dannon)	1 cup	240	11	3
Banana, Custard Style (Yoplait)	6 oz	190	19	4
Blueberry (Dannon)	1 cup	240	11	3
Blueberry (Yoplait)	6 oz	190	14	3
Boysenberry (Dannon)	1 cup	240	11	3
Cherry (Dannon)	1 cup	240	11	3
Coffee, low-fat	1 cup	194	14	3
Coffee (Dannon)	1 cup	200	14	3
Dutch Apple (Dannon)	1 cup	240	11	3
Exotic Fruit (Dannon)	1 cup	240	11	3
Fruit flavors, low-fat	1 cup	225	12	3
Lemon (Dannon)	1 cup	200	14	3
Mixed Berries (Dannon)	1 cup	240	11	3
Mixed Berries (Dannon)	4.4 oz	130	14	2
Mixed Berries (Dannon Hearty Nuts & Raisins)	1 cup	260	10	3
Orchard Fruit (Dannon Hearty Nuts & Raisins)	1 cup	260	10	3
Peach (Dannon)	1 cup	240	11	3
Piña Colada (Dannon)	1 cup	240	11	3

Product	Portion	Calories	Percent Calories from Fat	Fat Grams
YOGURT				
Plain, Whole (Colombo)	1 cup	150	42	7
Plain, Lite (Colombo)	1 cup	110	0	0
Plain, Lowfat (Dannon)	1 cup	140	26	4
Plain, Nonfat (Dannon)	1 cup	110	0	0
Raspberry (Dannon)	1 cup	240	11	3
Raspberry (Dannon)	4.4 oz	130	14	2
Raspberry (Yoplait 150)	6 oz	150	0	0
Raspberry, Custard Style (Yoplait)	6 oz	190	19	4
Strawberry (Dannon)	1 cup	240	11	3
Strawberry (Yoplait 150)	6 oz	150	0	0
Strawberry Banana (Dannon)	1 cup	240	11	3
Strawberry Banana (Yoplait 150)	6 oz	150	0	0
Vanilla, low-fat	1 cup	194	14	3
Vanilla (Dannon)	1 cup	200	14	3
Vanilla (Dannon Hearty Nuts & Raisins)	1 cup	270	17	5
YOGURT DRINKS (DAN' UP)				
Exotic Fruit	1 cup	190	19	4
Mixed Berries	1 cup	190	19	4

Product	Portion	Calories	Percent Calories from Fat	Fat Grams

YOGURT

YOGURT DRINKS (DAN' UP)

Product	Portion	Calories	Percent Calories from Fat	Fat Grams
Raspberry	1 cup	190	19	4
Strawberry	1 cup	190	19	4
Strawberry Banana	1 cup	190	19	4

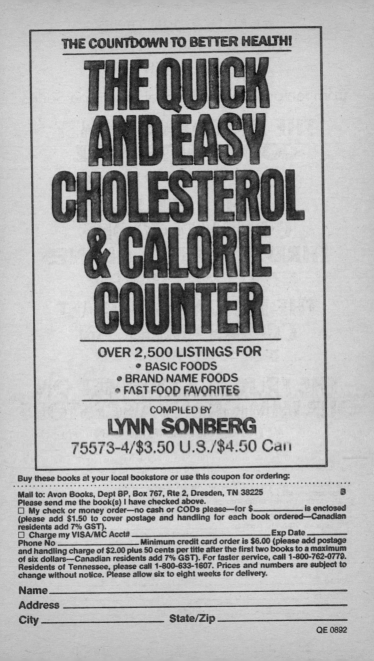

THE COUNTDOWN TO BETTER HEALTH!

THE QUICK AND EASY CHOLESTEROL & CALORIE COUNTER

OVER 2,500 LISTINGS FOR
- BASIC FOODS
- BRAND NAME FOODS
- FAST FOOD FAVORITES

COMPILED BY

LYNN SONBERG

75573-4/$3.50 U.S./$4.50 Can

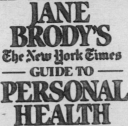